STplace
OF HEALTH

With Love,
Glori

MYplace

FOR BIBLE STUDY

D1065750

Published by First Place for Health
Galveston, Texas, USA
www.firstplaceforhealth.com
Printed in the USA

ISBN: 978-1-942425-34-2

CONTENTS

MY PLACE FOR BIBLE STUDY
Beyond Free

FOREWORD

I was introduced to First Place for Health in 1993 by my mother-in-law, who had great concern for the welfare of her grandchildren. I was overweight and overwrought! God used that first Bible study to start me on my journey to health, wellness, and a life of balance.

Our desire at First Place for Health is for you to begin that same journey. We want you to experience the freedom that comes from an intimate relationship with Jesus Christ and witness His love for you through reading your Bible and through prayer. To this end, we have designed each day's study (which will take about fifteen to twenty minutes to complete) to help you discover the deep truths of the Bible. Also included is a weekly Bible memory verse to help you hide God's Word in your heart. As you start focusing on these truths, God will begin a great work in you.

At the beginning of Jesus' ministry, when He was teaching from the book of Isaiah, He said to the people, "The Spirit of the Lord is on me, because he has anointed me to preach good news to the poor. He has sent me to proclaim freedom for the prisoners and recovery of sight for the blind, to release the oppressed, to proclaim the year of the Lord's favor" (Luke 4:18–19). Jesus came to set us free—whether that is from the chains of compulsivity, addiction, gluttony, overeating, undereating, or just plain unbelief. It is our prayer that He will bring freedom to your heart so you may experience abundant life.

God bless you as you begin this journey toward a life of liberty.

Vicki Heath, First Place for Health National Director

ABOUT THE AUTHOR

A popular speaker and writer, Gari Meacham travels the globe speaking at conferences, retreats, and events for women. Her highly acclaimed books, workbooks, and DVD series *Spirit Hunger*, *Watershed Moments*, and *Truly Fed* are used in book groups and churches across the country. Gari is President and Founder of The Vine—a ministry to orphans and widows in Uganda, and SHINE—a trendy YouTube show she hosts with her daughter Ally. She is married to former New York Yankee Bobby Meacham, and together they have three children. Bobby and Gari have been in professional baseball for more than thirty years and call Houston their home.

ABOUT THE CONTRIBUTOR

Lisa Lewis, who provided the menus and recipes in this study, is the author of *Healthy Happy Cooking* and *Deliciously Happy*. Lisa's cooking skills have been a part of First Place for Health wellness weeks and other events for many years. She provided recipes for fourteen of the First Place for Health Bible studies and is a contributing author in *Better Together* and *Healthy Holiday Living*. She partners with community networks, including the Real Food Project, to bring healthy cooking classes to underserved areas. She is dedicated to bringing people together around the dinner table with healthy, delicious meals that are easy to prepare. Lisa lives in Galveston and is married to John. They have three children: Tal, Hunter, and Harper. Visit www.healthyhappycook.com for more delicious inspiration.

INTRODUCTION

First Place for Health is a Christ-centered health program that emphasizes balance in the physical, mental, emotional, and spiritual areas of life. The First Place for Health program is meant to be a daily process. As we learn to keep Christ first in our lives, we will find that He is the One who satisfies our hunger and our every need.

This Bible study is designed to be used in conjunction with the First Place for Health program but can be beneficial for anyone interested in obtaining a balanced lifestyle. The Bible study has been created in a seven-day format, with the last two days reserved for reflection on the material studied. Keep in mind that the ultimate goal of studying the Bible is not only for knowledge but also for application and a changed life. Don't feel anxious if you can't seem to find the correct answer. Many times, the Word will speak differently to different people, depending on where they are in their walk with God and the season of life they are experiencing. Be prepared to discuss with your fellow First Place for Health members what you learned that week through your study.

There are some additional components included with this study that will be helpful as you pursue the goal of giving Christ first place in every area of your life:

○ **Leader Discussion Guide:** This discussion guide is provided to help the First Place for Health leader guide a group through this Bible study. It includes ideas for facilitating a First Place for Health class discussion for each week of the Bible study.

○ **Jump Start Menus and Recipes:** There are seven days of meals, and all are interchangeable. Each day totals 1,300 to 1,400 calories. Instructions are given for those who need more calories.

○ **Steps for Spiritual Growth:** This section will provide you with some basic tips for how memorize Scripture and make it a part of your life, establish a quiet time with God each day, and share your faith with others..

○ **First Place for Health Member Survey:** Fill this out and bring it to your first meeting. This information will help your leader know your interests and talents.

○ **Personal Weight and Measurement Record:** Use this form to keep a record of your weight loss. Record any loss or gain on the chart after the weigh-in at each week's meeting.

- **Weekly Prayer Partner Forms:** Fill out this form before class and place it into a basket during the class meeting. After class, you will draw out a prayer request form, and this will be your prayer partner for the week. Try to call or email the person sometime before the next class meeting to encourage that person.

- **100-Mile Club:** A worthy goal we encourage is for you to complete 100 miles of exercise during your twelve weeks in First Place for Health. There are many activities listed on pages 265-266 that count toward your goal of 100 miles.

- **Live It Trackers:** Your Live It Tracker is to be completed at home and turned in to your leader at your weekly First Place for Health meeting. The Tracker is designed to help you practice mindfulness and stay accountable with regard to your eating and exercise habits.

WEEK ONE: FREEDOM VERSUS DIETING

SCRIPTURE MEMORY VERSE

It is for freedom that Christ has set us free. Stand firm, then, and do not let yourselves be burdened again by a yoke of slavery. **Galatians 5:1**

There's nothing worse than achieving a goal, then crawling back to where you were (or worse) before the achievement. Welcome to the world of dieting. I listen to countless tales of victory, glory, pants zipping, control-stomping joy after a successful season of dieting. But soon, those same stomps of glory become a shameful walk of defeat. Why?

The answer lies in the truth that dieting and mastering control of every bite entering our mouths isn't the goal...freedom is. Anyone can follow a well-laid plan and lose weight. If you're strict enough and diligent enough—pounds will drop. But what happens weeks after your goal is met? How do you handle the mental strain of perfection? How do you establish a relationship with food wherein it's not the enemy, but rather, an ally in the pursuit of knowing the depths of God?

I've been free from food compulsion for over thirty years, and I credit food for teaching me some of my most profound life lessons. Lessons of trust, obedience, self-control, belief, hope, tenacity, endurance, and commitment emerged as "food" lessons became "kingdom" lessons. For all of us who've struggled to wrap our minds around what it means to be truly free, the scripture is clear...it is for FREEDOM that Christ has set us free. Why are we tempted to crawl back to a comfy perch in prison? Galatians 5:1 offers a past-tense promise with a present tense punch. Jesus set us free, so we could live in freedom...now. It says we must stand our ground and not be burdened again by any form of slavery. That means yo-yo dieting, scale obsession, body bashing, binge eating, overeating, calorie compulsion, and a perpetual diet mindset.

In the weeks ahead we'll study and pray, binding ourselves to two staunch beliefs. First, freedom is real because Jesus offered it. He wouldn't have teased us with it if it weren't true. Second, freedom is neither perfection nor permission.

Many of you bravely walked the pages of my first book called *Be Free*. We climbed the steep hills of freedom, establishing safe perimeters of hope and tenacious belief as we ascended higher in our knowledge and understanding of our Savior's mandate. In *Beyond Free* we'll travel the lush plateaus of mature assurance. We'll study the power of obedience and what holds us in the chains of defeat. *Beyond Free* isn't a place we arrive when we've studied hard enough and mastered self-control. Freedom can never be contained by the measures of man-made achievement. It's the brilliant knowledge that we can't go back—we won't go back—to lesser ways. It's the revelation that God's kingdom is vast and inviting, and anything that keeps us from its fullness and pleasure must go.

It's my joy to journey with you for the next twelve weeks. We'll lock arms and travel this freedom terrain together. We'll confidently stake our claim at the top of our climb: "It is for freedom that Christ has set me free...." Nothing else will do.

—— DAY 1: IT'S NOT ABOUT WILLPOWER

Lord Jesus, as I seek to understand the true nature of freedom, I realize it's a concept that seems hard to grasp. Teach me to understand that as I know truth, I'll be set free. Amen.

If you wander the shelves of any bookstore, you'll see more books on dieting, health, and exercise than any other topic combined. According to Marketdata Enterprises, Americans spend more than $60 billion dollars annually trying to lose weight.[1] Yet, obesity rates have skyrocketed, and we've never been more food and weight obsessed. What's going on?

Perhaps the problem is we're asking the wrong question and pursuing the wrong outcome. What if the question weren't "How can I lose weight?" but rather, "How can I be free?" What if we let Jesus into the darkest closets of habits and defeat? What if we re-wrote the script on how we view food consumption and the ever-elusive golden ring of weight loss? Many people think if they had more willpower, they'd master their appetites and overcome the bulging battle. But more willpower is not the secret. Not even close.

Freedom has little to do with our will and nothing to do with our power. My will wants to eat healthy but also wants to devour four maple glazed donuts. My power stops at the lure to fill myself with food when I'm actually hungry for God. Willpower is mustering up our own strength to make good choices. Nothing wrong with that, except over the course of time our limited ability wanes as the temptation towards complacency (I'm sick of healthy food—give
me a bag of chips.), deception (I deserve to eat or drink whatever I want. I earned it.) and defeat (What's the use? Nothing I do seems to last.) sets in. Without the power of God—willpower is a toy tugboat thrashed in the waves of defeat. So, if it's not about willpower, then what is it about?

Please turn to Genesis 3 and read verses 1-7. What did the serpent ask Eve in verse 1?

_____

_____

I know you may be familiar with these verses, but you're going to see something remarkable as we work through this lesson. Verses 2-5 showcase the typical willpower battle. We know the right thing to do (vs. 2-3), but then the truth gets twisted, and what we know becomes a rationalized heap of confusion. How does Satan twist the truth in verses 4-5?

_____

_____

_____

It's interesting that the very first battle between our will and the will of God was centered around food. The enemy used something harmless and good to seduce us into destruction. What three things did Eve's "willpower" rationalize as she considered eating something she knew would cause her harm (vs. 6)?

_____

_____

_____

To God it's rarely about the food; it's about the wisdom. We attach meaning to certain types of food as if sugar were evil and bread were bad. Interestingly, when the prophet Isaiah described the coming Messiah, he said he'd eat curds (butter) and honey (Isaiah 7:15) Hardly a combo we'd see on a popular diet! When God told Adam and Eve which trees they could eat from and the one they couldn't, he was protecting their lives from the dark world of sin, not giving them a good food/bad

food check list. After eating from the forbidden tree, what kind of leaves did they use to cover themselves when they realized they were naked (vs. 7)?

_____

_____

_____

Most scholars don't think the tree Eve picked from was an apple tree like our culture suggests. As a matter of fact, it's more likely it was a fig tree. Figs are common in that region of the world, and the fact they grabbed fig leaves indicates they were standing near a fig tree!

Now turn to Matthew 21:18-22 and describe the tree Jesus sees as they walked towards Jerusalem.

_____

_____

_____

_____

Jesus saw the leaves on this tree and moved towards it because he was hungry. This is one of the few times we see the humanity of God nestled within the glory of God. This fig tree had the chance of a lifetime: to feed and nourish the Savior, and yet, it had no real fruit. Jesus used this as a teaching moment for his disciples and for all of us for centuries to come. When Jesus saw there were no figs on the tree, he cursed the tree and it withered at once. Write what Jesus said to his shocked disciples below (vs. 21-22)?

_____

_____

_____

_____

Hidden in these verses is a new mandate on willpower and sin. Bible history believes that Jesus was crucified just a few yards away from this withered fig tree. In his proclamation against a fake fig tree promising nourishment, he screamed, "Never again will you, fig tree, offer a false fruit. Never again will you deceive people into thinking what you offer is real." In this symbolic moment Jesus spoke straight to the heartache of sin.

I think the disciples thought Jesus was losing his mind! Why scream like a mad man at a fig tree? Why not calmly walk to a café and get some bread? The disciples were fixated on the fact the tree withered, while Jesus was focused on something bigger... faith.

What does Jesus say will happen if we truly have faith and don't doubt (vs. 21)?

_____

_____

_____

Jesus was conquering more than a fig tree that day; he was taking care of what started in the garden at the beginning of time. The first mention of a fig tree is the leaves Adam and Eve used to cover their shame. Now, just a few yards from a withered fig tree Jesus died on the cross to overcome sin, poor choices, failed willpower, and shame. He offered more than a lame fig tree promising fulfillment and more than the power of our will to make good choices.

What kind of "fig leaves" do you use to cover your shame? Do you stay busy or keep people at bay? Are you overly critical or a person addicted to approval? Perhaps shame plays out in how you feel towards your body or the scars from a tainted past. Explain below.

_____

_____

_____

_____

_____

The good thing about fig leaves is they're a temporary covering that we've tried to hold in place. Jesus replaces our fig leaves with a different kind of clothing. Read Isaiah 61:10 and describe the robe that will clothe us.

_____

_____

_____

_____

Now turn to Luke 15:20-24 and note what kind of robe the Father placed on the son.

_____

_____

_____

Finally, let's look at Jesus' robe in Revelation 19:11-16. Please read these verses twice and really let them settle. What invigorates you in these verses?

_____

_____

_____

Jesus, I love the secret treasures of your Word. What began at a fig tree in the garden ended at the foot of your cross. Give me bold faith to believe. Amen.

—— DAY 2: WHAT'S WRONG WITH DIETING?

Lord, I'm used to thinking with a diet mentality. I'm not sure what a free mentality is. Please open my mind to your truth today as I study. Amen.

I tend to be picky about who gives me advice. I listen respectively to everyone, but I trust those who've walked in the shoes I'm walking in. These companions have endured similar heartache or bravely slain similar giants. That's the comfort we have together in Beyond Free. I never teach what I haven't lived. You can trust the stories and insight I share have all come with scars. As we pursue the gift of freedom, I need you to know who I am and why I'm passionate about your freedom.

When I was nine years old my father was in a tragic car accident that left him paralyzed from the neck down. Our family spiraled into chaos as mom turned to alcohol for relief, and I shouldered the weight of raising my younger siblings who were six and three years old. By the time I got to college certain patterns formed in my behaviors with food. It was my secret comfort and delight. I remember saying to a yellow bag of Lay's Potato Chips, "You will never hurt or fail me." But hurt and fail it did.

My first two years of college are a blur of binging, self-hatred, and the horrible realization that I simply couldn't stop eating. I gained so much weight that giant sweat pants and baggy tops were all I could wear. Eventually I was so disgusted that I resolved (for the umpteenth time) to diet my body into submission. Somehow, I mustered the strength to follow a diet perfectly, and the pounds began to melt away. I was elated—but after a year and a half of diet perfection I became obsessed with the regiment of harsh dieting and dangerously substituted one compulsion for another. Deep in the throes of anorexia, I contemplated taking my life as I saw no way out of the food prison I languished in. In desperation I cried out to Jesus to save me. I wasn't even sure he was real, but immediately things began to change. My diet mentality was replaced with a freedom mindset. It took time to understand and mature (which we'll do together in this book), but the difference was profound.

I want you to respond to this question as honestly as you can. Why is dieting easier than pursuing freedom?

Perhaps you noted that dieting is something we can master while freedom is something only the Master can give. Let's look at three core beliefs about dieting and true freedom.

Dieting is temporary; freedom is a gift for life.

Turn to John 8 and read verses 31-36. What is the promise Jesus made to the people who believed in Him?

_____

_____

Jesus made it clear that if we abide (live in, breathe in, soak in) his Word, then we are truly disciples, and we will know truth and that truth will set us free. The problem is sometimes we forget to abide. We stop in periodically or wink as we rush out the door. What does abiding with Jesus mean to you, and how does that impact your quest for freedom when it comes to food?

_____

_____

_____

Diets have a start and a stop. They have temporary boundaries, while freedom is a gift that matures over a lifetime. The minute you ask Jesus to set you free rather than to merely lose a set amount of weight, you've opened the door to freedom.

Dieting is carnal, freedom is spiritual.

Turn to Colossians 2 and read verses 20-23. What does the apostle Paul emphasize in verse 23?

_____

_____

_____

How does dieting fit into this description?

_____

_____

_____

As the scripture explains, diets rely on severe treatment of the body over a course of time, which Paul notes is of little value against fleshly indulgence. Most of our issues with food are spiritual in nature, and the answer lies in a spiritual quest for freedom not a fleshly quest to simply zip up skinny jeans. In verse 20 Paul is inviting us to leave the elementary principles of the world for something deeper that pulses with new life.

Diets are a band-aid; freedom is a life change.

Please turn to Romans 8:11-17. Write verse 13 below.

_____

_____

_____

What is the fear Paul mentions in verse 15? What does that fear look like to you?

_____

_____

_____

_____

Read Psalm 119:45 out loud three times as it seeps down into your spirit: "I will walk about in freedom, for I have sought out your precepts."

Father, you promise freedom rather than the shallow act of dieting. We don't want a band-aid or merely weight loss...we want a deeper understanding of you. Amen.

—— DAY 3: WHY SLAVERY SOMETIMES LOOKS GOOD

Lord, you offer freedom from destruction and hope for weary resolve. I never want to return to the things that held me captive. Amen.

The problem with freedom is it's hard to define. The dictionary explains it as "the power or right to act, speak, or think as one wants without hindrance or restraint." This is a good place to start. Imagine the freedom Jesus promises: enabling us to act, speak, and think without hindrance or restraint. Dream with me for a moment. Let's picture ourselves eating well without hindrance. We're consistently enjoying the healthy and sane way we approach food. We're acting, speaking, and thinking in ways that are true and empowering. We're free.

I've been asked by radio hosts and groups at gatherings if my freedom is real. Because we live in a world where people claim to be one thing and secretly living like another, I take my response seriously. My answer is always the same, "As real as the sky is blue."

I'll never forget the moment I realized I was free. I was kneeling on the orange shag carpet of my in-laws' home, praying about a host of things, when a wave of revelation washed over me and the thrill of freedom tingled from my head to my toes. I belted out this sentence to my startled husband Bobby, "I want to pinch myself! It's real...I'm truly set free!" Prior to our trip to visit his parents, I'd been grappling with issues of bondage to food. Former ways of thinking and beating myself up were again lodging in my soul. Even though I'd experienced moments of freedom, the entire package had not yet been revealed. We'll talk more about that in our lesson tomorrow, but for today I want us to look at why we sit on the fence of freedom and slavery. What keeps us one foot in and one foot out?

Please turn to Exodus 15:22-27. Note that immediately following their passage through the Red Sea, the Israelites were prone to grumble. Describe what happened in the Desert of Shur below.

How did the Lord describe himself in verse 26? Why is this an important name for God as we pursue freedom?

Interestingly, the Israelites moved from the wilderness of Shur to camp in the beauty of Elim. Although they only stayed there for a short time, Elim was lush with twelve springs of water and seventy date palms. The fact the exact numbers of springs and trees were recorded is significant. In the Bible the number twelve represents faith. God chose twelve tribes to deliver his message in the Old Testament and twelve disciples in the New Testament. The number seventy is a combination of perfection (7) and completeness (10). Moses took seventy elders to the top of Mount Sinai to worship and hear from God (Exodus 24), and Jesus sent seventy disciples out on the first gospel mission to preach the good news. Tucked in this short and often forgotten verse we've studied is a secret path to God's future plan. On your road to freedom, it may feel as though you camp in the wilderness, with dry and dreary places that make you question your resolve to move to new lands and new landscapes.

Although some weeks feel like wilderness, God also leads us to Elim: spots where living water flows freely, and the food and shade of special trees are a delight.

Reflect on your current state with food, eating, and freedom. Are you in a wilderness or a camp like Elim? Why?

_____

_____

_____

_____

Read Exodus 16:1-3. Note the name of the next place the Israelites camped. How does the name of where they camped describe the condition of their hearts?

_____

_____

_____

_____

It's no accident they camped in the wilderness of Sin. Talk about symbolic names and places! In two short months the thrill of being free was reduced to the pleasure of eating meat. I can just hear their campfire discussions. "Wow...I really miss the taste of tender roast and biscuits. And what about the garlic and onions we added for flavor?" This is proof the lure of our taste buds and physical desires can often outweigh our longing to be free. In those moments the Israelites forgot how cruel slavery was—and at times, so do we.

Check the circles below that relate to your relationship with food:

- O I work hard all day. I deserve to eat what I want whenever I want to.
- O Tomorrow's a new day. I'll start a fresh diet after this meal or binge.
- O It could be worse. I could be struggling with alcohol, sex, or drugs.
- O I come from a heritage of big eaters. It's just the way I am.
- O God doesn't care about my body and eating habits. He has bigger things to care about.
- O Nothing I do seems to change my weight, so I might as well eat as much as I want.
- O Saying no to food is rude. I must eat everything I'm given.
- O I don't care how I'll feel later. I want this food now.

God has used food, both throughout history and now, to teach us obedience and trust. On Day 1 we noted how food was part of the first human temptation with Adam and Eve. Here we see it as part of the first human exodus towards freedom. And Jesus gave us the New Testament freedom cry (Matthew 4:4) while quoting the text from Deuteronomy 8:3 while hungry in the wilderness: "...man does not live on bread alone but on every word that comes from the mouth of the Lord."

Read God's response to Moses in Exodus 16:4 after he prayed about the people's complaint. Write God's words to Moses below and circle the word test.

_____

_____

_____

Two themes are at work in this passage that we must digest. First, God always provides what we need. ALWAYS. I've been known to mutter under my breath, "But he didn't provide what I wanted," as if that discounts the provision God did bring. What we want is often different than what we need. Mature men and women learn to be content regardless of the outcome.

Second, there will be tests. Ugh! I hate tests. In school I was never good at them, and in life I try to avoid them. But to God, tests are a chance to show off our love. A chance to prove that we've learned from the things we've lived and that we're ready to move on to something fresh and new. Ultimately, a test is a chance to pass not fail, and God is a teacher who allows retakes for those fully committed to trying their best.

Bible scholars note the number of quails God provided filled football fields. Thousands and thousands of quails daily! That's enough meat for a lifetime. I don't think one Israelite complained about meat after that first whining session because God took them to a different land. No use moaning about meat and potatoes when new life is promised ahead.

Father, I see a glimpse of new life before me. Thank you for the chance to pass your tests. Amen.

—— DAY 4: FREEDOM ON AN ORANGE SHAG CARPET
Jesus, help me to hear the truth about my habits and behaviors. I don't want to hide or be ignorant. I want to be free. Amen.

Yesterday I promised to explain more about what happened on the orange shag carpet at my in-laws' home. It's a story I love to re-tell because some moments completely change the way we think and behave. This was one of those moments.

Before we left our home in New Jersey to visit Bobby's parents in California, I picked up a small, plain book from our local Christian bookstore. I'd run there in a hurry after beating myself up in my closet while trying to fit into clothes after the birth of our second child. Given my struggles with overeating and undereating, the mental fatigue of self-hatred was pushing my limits. I figured that surely, in the history of mankind, someone must have written a book on how to manage the mental and physical strain of dieting from a Christ-like perspective. Had I seen any of First Place for Health's material (which this small store didn't have), I would have consumed it, but much to my disappointment there were only three books that dealt with food issues, and two of those books were strict dieting guidelines. Goodness knows that wasn't what I was looking for. I spotted a book with the title The Diet Alternative by Diane Hampton, and I snatched it up. I don't remember much about that book, but one concept she explained rocked my world. She framed our struggles with overeating as gluttony and talked about it as a sin problem rather than a discipline problem. Whoa!

In Be Free I shared how gluttony is defined as someone habitually eating and drinking in a greedy and voracious way. I still didn't see how that fit into my patterns of food obsession until I searched the Bible to see if that description made sense.

Please turn to Proverbs 23: 19-21. What does the Bible say about gluttony?

_____

It's interesting to note the Bible connects gluttons with drunkards. For any of us tempted to think obsession with food is not as dangerous as alcohol, think again. God says both will end up poor and drowsy. Poor in the sense of missing out on abundant freedom and fruit of the Spirit, and drowsy in that our minds aren't sharp and alert when they're always thinking about what we'll eat or drink next.
Read 1 Thessalonians 5: 4-11. How does the Apostle Paul warn us in verse 6?

_____

_____

_____

Although Paul is talking about the "Day of the Lord" and his return, he's also giving us a mandate for life until he comes. He reminds us to be alert and sober, so we won't miss a minute of his promises and purpose while we're here on earth. If I'm honest, I admit a good portion of my adulthood was wasted being obsessed with food—what I would eat, what I wouldn't eat—chasing my tail in circles. It wasn't until I realized I was dealing with gluttony, not my lack of control or ability to over-control, that I began to get free.

Sitting on the orange shag carpet I put gluttony together with sin for the first time. I was confused by the word sin, and thought it was each individual thing I did wrong. I was always waiting for a back-hand slap from God with a smirk of disappointment. I'd also been taught as a child that sins have categories, and some sins are so bad you can never recover from them. The brilliant preacher Oswald Chambers described sin as "deliberate and emphatic independence of God."[2] Within that definition I began to see how my behavior with food is different from a disease or the life-time sentence of walking a tightrope of compulsion.

Describe how your eating patterns may be independent of God. Are you deliberately holding on to them in a defensive way?

_____

_____

_____

One of the positive things about sin is we have a Savior who has defeated it. I love how Jesus takes the impossible parts of our lives and paints a whole new canvas. Turn to Isaiah 57 and read verses 14-15. Write verse 14 below.

_____

_____

In the previous verses Isaiah warned about the dangers of trusting idols (anything that contradicts or ignores the rightful place of God) for security and help. He instructed the people to build and prepare the road and remove any obstacles in the way. In Breaking Free Beth Moore explains that in ancient times kings would visit villages. To make it safely, villagers would have to remove any rocks or obstacles on the roadway. If the king tried to come but the obstacles weren't removed, the king moved on from the village to visit somewhere else.

What obstacles do you need to remove from your life so the King can have full access?

_____

_____

_____

Verse 15 shows the beauty of our King, who longs for the obstacles to be removed so he can revive those with a contrite heart. We may have never considered our behavior with food to be gluttony or sin or an obstacle to be removed for the King to have full access. We may have just thought we were big eaters, were low on self-control, or were lovers of certain types of food. My prayer is you'll have your own "shag carpet" moment when you realize the joy of confession and the realization that you can be truly free.

Turn back to Isaiah 57 and read verses 18-19 carefully. What is God promising to those who come to him with a broken and tender heart?

_____
_____
_____
_____

At this point you might be thinking, "Okay, Gari, I want an orange shag carpet moment, and I understand my independence and gluttonous behavior towards food—but what did you do next? What are my next steps towards freedom?" If I were with you right now, I'd kiss your cheek and say, "Take a breath. This isn't some quick fix or flimsy faith walk. You're going to get there, and He'll show you how." Tomorrow we'll look at one of our greatest assets as we trust our God for freedom.

Lord, I confess that I've held on to my behavior with food in an independent way. I lay it at your feet now. Amen

—— DAY 5: THE POWER OF PATIENCE
Lord, help me to be patient with myself as I learn about freedom. This isn't a race, it's a saunter of deliverance and hope. Amen.

Few things are as irritating as those requiring patience. Waiting in lines, waiting in traffic, waiting at the Department of Motor Vehicles office. I can tangibly feel the tension! In these situations, we typically trudge through knowing we must, but the pursuit of freedom is different. It takes patience to get to our new way of behaving, but the journey is anything but a trudge. It's a freedom walk that allows us to peacefully take in the scenery as we travel.

Please turn to James 1:4 and write the result of patience below.

_____

_____

_____

Some translations use the words perseverance or endurance, and although I like these words—they make me tired. Patience revs me up. Perhaps because Paul used it so many times in his writings to clarify gentleness, steadfastness, and kindness. As we're patient and committed to freedom, we'll be steadfast in our pursuit and kind to ourselves when we struggle. No longer under the whip of diet perfection, we are empowered to behave differently.

In *My Utmost for His Highest* Chambers talks about the "careless" areas of our lives. The areas that aren't blatantly hideous but have the undertone of a careless afterthought. He writes, "We should have no carelessness about us, either in the way we worship God or even in the way we eat and drink. Not only must our relationship to God be right, but the outward expression of that relationship must also be right."[3]

Most of us are decent men and women trying to do the right things. We're teachers, mothers, fathers, doctors, ministry leaders, and executives who care about people and the world we live in. But once again, it's not about being good—it's about being free. God is a master surgeon who will come back to that one hidden spot, over and over again, until what harms us is removed. Chambers goes on to say, "And He never tires of bringing us back to that one point until we learn the lesson, because His purpose is to produce the finished product. It may be a problem with our impulsive nature, and with persistent patience, God brings us back to that one point. Or the problem may be our idle and wandering thinking, or our independent nature and self-interest. God is trying to impress upon us the one thing that is not entirely right in our lives."

For me, that one area not completely right was food. God patiently pried open the door I'd sealed shut. Can you explain your area of carelessness? Is there one (or more) areas that God keeps bringing you back to, but you don't seem to change?

_____

_____

_____

Once we're free from compulsion with food, we move beyond free to new areas of exploration and depth. The Holy Spirit will continue to reveal the careless corners of our lives that hold dust or cobwebs. Why? Because he loves us too much

to allow any behaviors that don't enable his purpose and power to live through us.

Please turn to 2 Corinthians 6 and read verses 3-10. Write the words he emphasizes in verse 6 below.

_____

_____

_____

Although we may not endure all the things Paul did in his lifetime, much of what he described we've been through. Verse 6 puts a blanket around the hardship with soothing words such as purity, understanding, patience, kindness, the Holy Spirit and sincere love. Although admitting and relinquishing the careless areas of our lives may be hard, the patience and kindness of our Surgeon is what carries us through.

Let's take this a step further. Let's acknowledge and heal these areas right now.

Step One: Meet with God this minute and explain the area(s) you keep coming back to. Habits, excused ways of behaving or reacting, careless attitudes towards things you're used to doing—confess whatever comes to mind. He already knows, but there's freedom in recognizing and admitting these areas to him.

Step Two: Right now, pray this prayer out loud, "Father, I've been careless with some areas of my life I now want changed. I can no longer excuse or rationalize this behavior. It must be dealt with and removed so I can function freely for your kingdom. I hand (write what you're praying about on the line) _____ to you so you can deal with it now.

Step Three: Praise God in your own personal way. It may be a song, a shout, a tear, or the words in a journal or margin of this book. Praise him that he is a God of freedom and that the areas that formerly were carelessly ignored are now under his protective care.

You may not feel any different, but I promise the air around you just shifted with your prayer and commitment. Tomorrow I'll offer some tangible ways to mark your freedom, but today let's close with the Psalms.

Please read Psalm 32:7 and write the verse below.

Lord, you are my hiding place. You surround me with songs of deliverance. Thank you for removing my careless places. Amen.

——— DAY 6: REFLECTION AND APPLICATION

Lord, as I try to comprehend a new way of approaching food, fill me with a super-natural capacity to understand. Your word says You will accomplish what concerns me. Amen.

It's one thing to talk about freedom and another to truly walk it out. I'm not only a visual learner—I'm an action learner. Research shows that if you tell someone

something, they will retain a portion of what you said. But if you walk with them through what you taught, offering tools and feedback...they change. Freedom always demands change, so we're going to do everything we can to have tools and encouragement in place.

As I was pursuing freedom in its beginning stages, and now in more mature stages, I've used a few tools I'm going to share with you today. They many seem ridiculous, but when you're face-to-face with stuffing your mouth with food you don't really want, it's good to have some tools ready for escape!

TOOL #1: In my first book *Truly Fed*, I mentioned a simple phrase that to this day, people refer to as one of their greatest tools towards change. When I was initially pursuing freedom, I'd slam up against moments that seemed impossible to overcome: moments of severe physical temptation or the mental temptation to circle back to poor choices or numb outlooks. I began to say a simple phrase that holds a spiritual power:

I don't do that anymore.

Some might say, "Why not a beautiful scripture or promise of strength?" There's a place for that tool and you'll see it below. But in the swirl of a moment, this phrase knocks the foam off the top of anything trying to derail our freedom. I wrote it on a paper plate and for months had it taped to my refrigerator. Now I use it to defend my thoughts when the enemy tries to make me do or respond in ways I've grown beyond.

TOOL #2: In the first scene of the popular TV drama *This Is Us* we see Kate, an overweight woman, reaching into her fridge. When she opens the door, we see sticky notes written and placed over birthday cake and various food items she wants to stay away from. Right away we love her because we all can relate! The problem with her strategy is boosting our willpower and dieting skills never translates to long-term freedom. What if you try this? Place sticky notes on the inside of your fridge, pantry, or cabinets that say: "It's not about the willpower to not eat. It's about the God-power to be spiritually full, active, and aware of His strength to overcome." Or our memory verse for this week: "It is for freedom that Christ has set us free. Stand firm, then, and do not let yourselves be burdened again by a yoke of slavery." (Galatians 5: 1)

TOOL #3: When I first began to write about freedom from eating behaviors, I conducted some personal research. I noticed the intensity to eat or the timeframe I stood contemplating a wrong choice totaled less than a minute. So, I began what I call the "Three Minute Escape." When you feel drawn to food in a compulsive way (not hungry but eating to smother or avoid feelings, to fill boredom, to fall back into habitual poor choices), escape either physically or mentally for three minutes. Three minutes is typically all you need to re-direct a poor choice. If you can change your physical surroundings—do! Instead of perching in the kitchen try these options: walk outside, walk around the neighborhood or down the street, look at birds or people or anything you don't ingest, sing and move to your favorite song on your playlist, go to your bathroom, or take a moment to praise God alone. You get the picture. Get out of the fridge, pantry, or cabinets and re-direct your mind. If you're at a restaurant or work and you're faced with a challenge, take three minutes and picture Psalm 23: "He makes me lie down in green pastures, he leads me beside quiet waters, he refreshes my soul." Often when I'm in tense situations, I recall a meadow on the ranch my grandparents owned in the Colorado mountains. I picture lying on a big quilt next to Jesus, looking up at the blue sky in complete peace. It only takes a moment of peace with Jesus to overcome a torrent of destruction.

Which of these tools might work for you? Write out your plan of action now so that in the moment, you're able to stand firmly.

_____

_____

_____

_____

Perhaps you can modify one of the tools or create your own based on your personality. Write your ideas below and share them with your group or a friend the next time you meet.

_____

_____

_____

_____

Jesus, don't let me diminish the power of simple re-directs in my life. You created my mind; you also have the power to change it. Amen.

—— DAY 7: REFLECTION AND APPLICATION
Father, I thank you today is a day I reflect on your concepts and deep love. I place my hand in yours to live this day fully. Amen.

On Day Four I shared that while kneeling on the orange shag carpet of Bobby's childhood bedroom, I had a moment of revelation. In one crisp moment I realized that I was free. That moment was defined with a profound assurance that what I was experiencing was real. The problem with such moments is we talk ourselves right out of them. "That didn't really happen." "I'm crazy to think I heard from God."

The reality is those moments are the milestones of our faith. And although I don't go around boasting of a plethora of moments (that cheapens them and makes them seem common), I do love to share them when I know they've been real. That shag carpet was the beginning of a story of freedom I'd share for decades to come. God has used that moment to encourage thousands of fellow sojourners on their own quest for freedom.

Is there a moment from God when you know you experienced wisdom or freedom concerning a situation? What was the situation and how has that moment impacted your life and the life of others?

_____

_____

_____

Reflect today on the power of revelation: the moments God reveals things personally to you through his Word, people, or any other creative way he chooses to speak.

Lord, your wisdom is the power of my life. Thank you for the stunning moments you reveal your mysteries to me. Amen.

Notes

1. Geoff Williams, "The Heavy Price of Losing Weight," U.S. News and World Report 2 Jan. 2013. https://money.usnews.com/money/personal-finance/articles/2013/01/02/the-heavy-price-of-losing-weight.
2. Oswald Chambers, My Utmost for His Highest (Grand Rapids, MI: Discovery House, 2018).
3. Oswald Chambers, ibid.

WEEK TWO: MY PERSONAL EXODUS

SCRIPTURE MEMORY VERSE
The Lord will fight for you while you keep silent. **Exodus 14:14**

To understand how to live beyond free, we must first understand how to get free. Many people admit their desire to be free from food struggles but have no idea how to get there. It's the illusive playground we can't seem to find. Thankfully, Jesus invites everyone to join in. The second book of the Bible is penned gold as even its name, Exodus, speaks of a freedom cry heard throughout the centuries

In all human history there's never been a story told as bold, challenging, and inspiring as the Exodus story. It involves wild faith and a supernatural God who not only changes the landscape but changes the hearts of those he sets free.

I've studied and taught the Bible for over three decades, and what I'm about to share this week still takes my breath away. As a matter of fact, I woke up at 4:30 this morning with these words singing in my soul, but I must warn you—freedom isn't for sissies. It's a mature call to live beyond our habits, our feelings, and our flesh. There's a life-changing reason you're doing this study—and a life-giving reason you're in a First Place group right now.

So, let me challenge you before we even begin. If you've been in groups for years and done multiple studies but seen little change or personal growth, I'm going to ask you to put your pen down right now and hear these words of truth.

This is your time. This is your season of unmeasurable growth and unprecedented freedom. Stop pretending and seek freedom as if your life depends on it. Don't let past defeat or a numb submission to the present define who you are. Rise up. Freedom is here.

—— DAY 1: THE STENCH OF OPPRESSION
Father, help me understand your redemptive heart. Lead me through my personal exodus. Amen.

When I began to get free from my issues with food, I didn't fully realize the bondage I was in until the chains began to fall. For so long I thought my struggles were minor, and I just needed more self-control. What I didn't fully realize was the spiritual implications of my choices and the debilitating lure of the enemy who enticed me to make them. When we're overcome with habits and feel as though we can never change—we're dealing with the effects of oppression. Simply put, oppression is prolonged cruel treatment or control. It's also described as mental pressure or distress.

I know some people think calling this struggle "oppression" might be a bit dramatic; after all, it's just food. But that's part of the problem. We need to realize anything that keeps us from the glory of God or from growing into the full identity he offers is oppressive. In our quest to live beyond free, we must rectify what keeps us stagnant and unlock the chains that hold us in place. To begin, let's identify areas we may feel oppressed. Check those that apply to you.

O   I struggle to make the right choices with food, even though I know better and want to. It leaves me feeling down and depressed.

O   I can't experience lasting change. I do well for a while on a new wave of resolve but eventually crawl back to my old ways.

O   My mind plays negative, harsh messages, and I can't seem to push the thoughts away.

O   The way I feel about myself plays into my relationships with family and friends. I tend to be someone who is overly harsh and critical or a slave to approval. Neither feels authentic.

O   If I'm honest, I don't understand why I keep struggling with the same things in life. I've prayed and begged God for direction and relief. Why doesn't he come through?

O   My past haunts me, even thought I know I'm forgiven. I can't seem to break free from what I've done or what's been done to me. It hinders my future and taints my hope.

If you identified with two or more of these items, you're most likely experiencing the weight of oppression. But rest assured—our God specializes in setting people free. No one would experience the joy of freedom if there weren't something they needed to be free from! Each day this week we'll lay out Freedom Principles based on the book of Exodus. These are the biblical principles that establish God's path towards freedom. Here's our freedom principle for today:

Freedom covers a multitude of incidents that build to a point of bondage. True freedom comes when oppression is revealed and destroyed.

Please turn to Exodus 1 and read verses 6-22. Describe what life was like for the Israelites living in Egypt.

_____

_____

_____

It's interesting to note that when Joseph was alive, the Egyptians respected the Israelites, and they were treated fairly, but after he died everything changed. (If you're not familiar with his story you can find it in Genesis 37.) The more the people of God flourished, the more the enemy felt threatened. It's the same for us today. When we begin to grow or see victory in our lives or move mightily in kingdom ways, the enemy gets scared! I'm thrilled by two midwives in this passage that weren't afraid to take a stand against the enemy. What were the names of these women (vs. 15)?

_____

_____

I love the fact their names were mentioned. It took a great deal of courage to do what they did, and any freedom story is filled with people just like them...and just like us. Can you imagine the conversations they had with Moses's mother Jochebod before and after she gave birth?

We know that Moses was saved from genocide and strategically ended up living with the Pharaoh who persecuted Moses's people. What happened in Exodus 2:11-14 that indicates the state of the Israelites' condition and the heart of Moses?

_____

_____

_____

How did God explain His perspective to Moses in Exodus 3:7-9?

_____

_____

Most translations use the word oppressed in verse 9, and rightly so. The Israelites were held down and afflicted by an enemy threatened by their presence. Unless we understand this principle in our own lives, we may remain under the oppressive thumb of an enemy who's afraid of our potential.

In our freedom principle today, we noted there are a multitude of incidents that build to a point of bondage. Let's explore this on a personal level. My book *Be Free* discusses "Life Frames." These are different time periods in our lives when certain destructive behaviors may have originated. My first memory of strange behavior with food was unwrapping the shiny silver wrapping on a stick of butter while standing behind a curtain. I was five years old and ate that butter like it was a candy bar. My mom found me behind the curtain and quickly began to tell me how bizarre I was. From that day forward, I sensed something was wrong with me, and I hid many of my behaviors (not behind curtains but in many other ways) as they warped into a confusing alliance with food.

Can you identify incidents that perhaps began innocently, but led you to a point of bondage? These may include attitudes or beliefs passed down from your family of origin, ways you pacify or numb yourself with food, or habits you've adopted that once seemed strange but now seem normal. Honestly reflect below.

_____

_____

_____

_____

In the book of Acts, Peter described the power of Jesus against oppression in a precise way. "You know of Jesus of Nazareth, how God anointed him with the Holy Spirit and with power, and how he went about doing good and healing all who were oppressed by the devil, for God was with Him" Acts 10:38 (NASB). It's the joy and pleasure of Jesus to do good towards you and to heal all oppression by bringing the presence of God into your habits, thoughts, behaviors, and sin.

Friends, you are on the eve of a great breakthrough. Identifying oppression and realizing its stench is the first step towards breaking free from it.

Jesus, I thank you that You went about doing good and healing the oppressed. Reveal things to me and heal me too. Amen.

—— DAY 2: THE REALITY OF BONDAGE

I often share the story of a man offered a new chance at life who refused to take it. He lived in a beaten down place in a dangerous neighborhood. His response to denying a chance to change was, "I may live in hell, but at least I know all the street names!" How often we excuse bondage because we're used to it or are afraid to let go of what we're accustomed to.

One of the challenging parts to the Exodus story is the Israelites lived in bondage for so long that even their misery was predictable and somewhat accepted. They cried to God for help but saw no real way out. Little did they know a small boy who'd been saved from the genocide would rise up and lead them from their pain.

The thing about freedom stories is they sound so magical once they're retold after the action plays out, but for those who've been major actors on freedom's stage, we know the fight for freedom isn't easy. It demands a price, or it wouldn't be so valuable. Yesterday we established our first Freedom Principle:

Freedom covers a multitude of incidents that build to a point of bondage. True freedom comes when oppression is revealed and destroyed.

Today we'll explore the second Freedom Principle:

Freedom requires some type of sacrifice and the belief that life can be different.

Turn to Exodus 3 and read verses 1-5. What was Moses's reaction to how God was calling him?

At first, Moses merely wanted to get a glimpse of something unusual...a burning bush that wasn't consumed. But from that bush God called out to Moses and the life of a quiet shepherd would never be the same.

Read vs. 10-14. What was Moses's response to God (vs. 11) and how did God respond to his fear?

Now read Exodus 4:1-5. What common item belonging to Moses did God use to show his power? Why do you think God chose this item?

We must remember that when God invites us to a calling He has planned for us, He will always provide a way for us to be successful. He doesn't call us to something He won't see us through. I know people who are scared to try new things or believe life can be different because they're afraid to fail. Moses was groomed his entire life for this moment. What if he stood at the burning bush and said, "You know what, God? This is too hard. I'm going to take my staff and head home."

Our Freedom Principle today explains that freedom demands a sacrifice. Sometimes that sacrifice is giving up the belief we're not strong enough to change. God does the miraculous, but He expects us to do the day-to-day, faithful things that usher the miraculous in.

What are some of the day-to-day faithful things you can do regarding food that can help set the stage for supernatural healing and freedom?

_____

_____

_____

The next thing we examine is one of the hardest realities in scripture. Sometimes, when you decide to do something about slavery, the situation may seem to get worse before it gets better.

Please read Exodus 5. What happened when Moses and Aaron asked Pharaoh for a three-day break in the wilderness?

_____

_____

_____

Notice they weren't asking for complete freedom, just a break to worship the Lord God. Pharaoh's reaction seemed to stun everyone, especially Moses and Aaron, who were only doing exactly what God had said to do. It's in these moments we must remember a few things about freedom and obedience. We can be doing exactly what we're supposed to do and still experience frustration and setbacks. It doesn't mean we're not on the right track; it only signals we're not in control of the track.

Moses, Aaron, and the Israelites didn't know that God was allowing the suffering to temporarily increase so the freedom would be more desirous and miraculous. They were used to suffering—that was clear—but when it became intolerable, it prepared them to move.

The question to ask ourselves is this: are we complacent with our bondage, or are we so tired of it we'll truly sacrifice for change?

Lord God, when I try to truly change, things get harder and I want to quit. Help me remember that a true exodus always demands a sacrifice. Amen.

──── DAY 3: WHAT IT COSTS TO BE FREE

Jesus, while freedom cost me nothing but belief and obedience, it cost You Your life. Thank You for this unspeakable gift. Amen.

In our quest to live Beyond Free, there's always a point of climax. A point of no return. A mandate that draws a line in the sand and dares trouble to broach it. Today's lesson is that line in the sand. We can talk about freedom, pray for freedom, and even pretend we're free—but we'll soon face a defining moment that demands proof. Either we're either willing to go all in or we sit on the fence watching those willing to get dirty and try.

This week we've defined our first two Freedom Principles as follows:

Freedom covers a multitude of incidents that build to a point of bondage. True freedom comes when oppression is revealed and destroyed.

Freedom requires some type of sacrifice and the belief life can be different.

Today we'll add a third principle to this list:

Freedom takes risks. We must be willing to risk who we are to be free.

Sometimes I wish there were an easier way. Several years ago, I taught a class on food issues. When we came to the week focused on freedom and obedience, a young woman raised her hand and exclaimed, "I thought this was about freedom!" When she heard that freedom demanded something from her, she walked out. Apparently, this woman thought she could be free without participating in her freedom!

Today we'll look at the cost of freedom and how we'll handle our point of no return. Please turn to Exodus 11 and read verses 1-6. How did the Lord assure Moses in verse 1, and what strange instruction did he give in verse 2?

_____

_____

_____

_____

Not only did Pharaoh finally let God's people leave; they got to take their oppressors' silver and gold along too! When we sacrifice to live free—God gives us supernatural favor and blessings we didn't even think to ask for. After nine horrible plagues the showdown came down to one symbolic, horrific event.

Please read Exodus 12:1-13. Describe how the Israelites were to place the blood of the lamb on the door.

_____

_____

_____

_____

Most movies depict this mark of blood as a red X, but scholars believe it looked more like a cross. One large mark horizontally and one vertically—symbolizing the ultimate freedom from death and sin. It didn't matter how messed up the family was or how far from God they'd been—if they were obedient to the mark of the cross, they were spared and free. No question. From this point on, every person of Hebrew descent understood that in place of their lives, another life would be sacrificed. This was God's plan of redemption unfolding first with the Passover lamb and finally with the Lamb of God—Jesus Christ.

God gave a few more interesting instructions in verses 8-10. How was the lamb to be prepared and eaten—and what other foods were to be eaten with it?

_____

_____

_____

At first glace we might wonder why God cares so much about the way food is prepared and the combination of what's eaten. In the case of the Passover Lamb, the lamb was roasted whole to symbolize unity and the unbroken body of the Lamb of God to come (John 19:36). Jewish commentators say the intestines were removed, washed clean, and replaced inside the lamb to show that nothing unclean remained in this sacrifice. The offering was perfect and holy in God's sight.

Why do you think God warned them about keeping leftovers? (vs. 10)

_____

_____

_____

In this prelude to the provision in the wilderness of manna and quail—God asked his people to trust him for what they needed tomorrow, not based on what they could save from the day before. It's interesting that God taught this lesson with food. Perhaps it's because our stomachs can make us moody and we don't like to restrain; we want to eat what we want when we want it. For those of us who like to pack a little snack no matter how long we'll be out or plan what we'll have for dinner before we've taken a bite of breakfast, trusting God for food provision can feel like a scary task. I have learned so much from my friends in Uganda, who eat breakfast and have no idea if dinner may come.

How did God say they should posture themselves to eat (vs. 11)?

_____

_____

Without lingering at a feast around the table, they were to be dressed and ready to move. They were to eat and then focus on how God was about to move. In our culture, food has risen to a popularity it wasn't created to withstand. Just flip through channels and you can find a show describing anything from cupcakes to kale—and don't get me started on YouTube and social media posts of perfectly "coifed" dishes dressed up like a family photo! I'm all for enjoying a good meal with friends and family—but God was speaking a message to these people (and to us) that would continue for forty years. Food is not the point—relationship with God is.

Ask yourself a probing question. How much of your day is spent thinking about food in an abnormal way?

_____

_____

I love the picture God paints in His instruction to the Israelites in verse 11. He's saying, "Be ready. Have your walking shoes and walking sticks ready to go. I'm on the move, and I don't want you to miss it by lingering around the food too long or worrying about what you'll eat tomorrow."

We'll end our time today with a detail from the Passover story that is rarely noticed. Read Exodus 12:22. What kind of branch was used to smear the blood of the lamb on the doors?

_____

_____

_____

Now turn to John 19:28-30. From what kind of branch was Jesus offered sour wine from minutes before dying on the cross?

_____

_____

In a stunning revelation of God's plan, the hyssop branch that smeared the life-saving blood of the lamb on the Israelites' doors was the same branch the Lamb of God drank from before uttering "It is finished."

Lord Jesus, You are the Lamb of God. May I never be satisfied with anything but You. Amen.

—— DAY 4: WAKING THE MIRACLE
Father, just when I think I don't know what's next, You show yourself in miraculous ways. Open my eyes to see. Amen.

When I began to experience freedom from my destructive behaviors with food, I noticed freedom was part obedience on my part and part miracle on God's. How else could I explain years of habits and poor choices changing before my eyes? I, the girl who thought Captain Crunch was one of the four food groups, now enjoyed carrots and salads. My taste buds grew up and left behind childish ways, and to this day, I know it's nothing short of a miracle.

Miracles are always born of circumstances that can't change unless God intervenes. I've been a part of several miracles in my life: the healing of my broken marriage, both of my daughters' redemption from violent men, and the freedom I've experienced with food. And they all have one thing in common: the hand of God moved as I was awakened in faith.

My friends, I'm going to invite you to something bold right now. You must wake up to see a miracle. No one sees a miracle if they are spiritually asleep or pridefully standing in the back murmuring, "Hah...it will never work." Right now, with our eyes wide open and our spirits alert, we are looking for our miracle.

Some might think calling healing from food behaviors a miracle is a bit theatrical. After all, isn't it just self-control laced with resolve? All I know is once I was lost, and now I'm found. I was blind but now I see. I believe that any time a man or woman turns from one behavior to another and is truly set free, it's a miracle.

Please turn to Ephesians 5:13-14 and write verse 14 below.

_____

_____

_____

Now turn to Hebrews 10:38-11:1 and write verse 11:1 below.

_____

_____

_____

These two explosive verses lay the foundation for experiencing personal breakthrough. The first tells us to wake up! When the Apostle Paul spoke these words to the church in Ephesus, he was referring to the prophet Isaiah who proclaimed, "But your dead will live, Lord; their bodies will rise—let those who dwell in the dust wake up and shout for joy..." (Isaiah 26:19). Paul spoke these words not to the dead, but to the living who needed to awaken to what God was doing in their midst as he transformed darkness.

The second thing we learn in Hebrews is faith isn't easy. How can we be assured of things we hope for and convicted about things we don't see? It's part mystery and part digging our heels in and determining nothing will stop where we want to go. It takes faith to have faith—and without it, we can't please God.

This week we've talked about three Freedom Principles, and today we'll add a new one to the list.

Freedom covers a multitude of incidents that build to a point of bondage. True freedom comes when oppression is revealed and destroyed.

Freedom requires some type of sacrifice and the belief that life can be different. Freedom takes risks. We must be willing to risk who we are to be free.

Freedom is miraculous and bears the handprint of God.

To better understand the waking of miracles and the handprint of God, we're heading back into the Exodus story.

Yesterday we learned the Israelites were ready to move. I can hear the songs and shouts of joy as over two million people walked out of a city that formerly held them in chains. The Lord led them away from the quickest route because it would have involved a bold battle with the Philistines, and frankly, they weren't ready for that. Instead, they settled by the sea. After a few days Pharaoh realized they weren't coming back and thought, "They are wandering aimlessly in the land; the wilderness has shut them in" (Exodus 14:3, NASB).

This is the launching point of miracles. Is there any area of your life where you feel as though you're wandering aimlessly? Ponder your work, parenting, marriage, relationships, finances, health, friendships or the lack of friendships, and overall purpose. Describe your feelings below.

_____

_____

_____

_____

This is our "hemmed in" point. But rest assured: this isn't the end of your story. As the Egyptians mounted their horses and chariots to go get their former slaves, Moses was alert to the assurance of God.

Read Exodus 14:10-16. If you were an Israelite on that beach, what would you shout as you heard the hoofs of your enemies' horses approach?

_____

_____

_____

_____

It's important to realize that seven days passed before the Red Sea parted. That's a long time to sit and stew in fear. One scholar noted that the people handled the crisis with these thoughts:

1.   Let's throw ourselves into the sea!
2.   Let's return to Egypt and go back to being slaves.
3.   Let's wage war on the Egyptians.
4.   Let's pray to God.

Sadly, praying to God was at the bottom of the list. Nonetheless, how did Moses handle their fear and what did he say to the people?

_____

_____

_____

Isn't it interesting that God wanted the people silent? I think their fear spread like fog, and as more people chanted negative worry, the more God needed their mouths to close. Moses tried to keep everyone calm and may have thought, "What in the world do I do next?"

Suddenly God reminded him of his staff—the same staff he saw turn into a serpent and change a river into blood. God instructed him to hold it out and watch a miracle of epic proportions. We know that the Red Sea was over 7,264 feet deep. Picture a wall of water like a skyscraper and a dry path lit by the interesting fish of the deep equipped with glowing lights. Friends, if God can do that for a bunch of fearful and murmuring former slaves, what can He do for you?

Lord God, Your power and desire to make a way out of no way thrills me. I know You will make a way for me. Amen.

—— DAY 5: WHEN THE ENEMY RUSHES IN

Lord, don't let me forget that when the enemy comes at me, You have already got me. Amen.

Just when we think we're ready for a victory lap something changes. We halt. We stumble. We struggle to make sense of what used to be clear. I used to be one of those Christians who glibly shouted, "If the enemy wants to challenge me...bring it on!" You know what? I never say that now because he always does. Why invite it? The enemy is a relentless hound sniffing out new ways to attack. Thankfully, freedom laughs at the wiles of the enemy. Next week we'll bravely study how to defeat that hound, but today we close out the Exodus story with a beautiful reminder. When God invites you to freedom—no enemy has the power to stop it.

Let's add our final Freedom Principle to the list we've been building this week.

- Freedom covers a multitude of incidents that build to a point of bondage. True freedom comes when oppression is revealed and destroyed.
- Freedom requires some type of sacrifice and the belief that life can be different.
- Freedom takes risks. We must be willing to risk who we are to be free.
- Freedom is miraculous and bears the handprint of God.
- The defeat of our enemy is final.

Please read Exodus 14:19-25. In what ways did God protect his people?

_____

_____

_____

The Living Bible describes God's first protective move like this: "Then the angel of God, who had been traveling in front of Israel's army, withdrew and went behind them. The pillar of cloud also moved from in front and stood behind them, coming between the armies of Egypt and Israel. Throughout the night the cloud brought darkness to the one side and light to the other side; so neither went near the other all night long (vs. 19-20).

After a celebration of hope, the enemy often tries to sneak back and recapture the freedom we've worked so hard to gain. The people had barely stopped praising God for their release when the enemy rolled in from a distance pursuing their excitement, their new belief, and their peace. I love how God's first protection on the shores of the Red Sea centers on darkness and light. The enemy couldn't find God's people because God was protecting them in His light. God's light still protects us today.

Read the following scriptures and note how light overcomes darkness.
John 1:5 _____
John 8:12 _____
1 John 1:5-6 _____

Here is the real question though. If we know He is the light and we long to stay in His presence, why do we settle for flashlights rather than His protective fire? I can't tell you the times I've reacted a way I regret, returned to an old way of viewing something I've moved beyond, or latched back onto a wave of insecurity. In these moments it's comforting to remember that God confuses the enemy. He keeps him in the dark while He continues to light our way.

What did the Egyptians say in response to their wheels jamming and their horses flinching (vs. 25)?

_____
_____

This is the truth we must remember. The Lord is fighting for us and against the enemy. Always. How do you typically react to the threat of the enemy? What's your go-to response?

- o Fear
- o Worry
- o Anger
- o Blame
- o Control
- o Avoidance
- o Prayer
- o Unflinching trust
- o Obedience regardless of circumstances

You're in good company if some of your checks are in the upper portion of this list. I can almost hear the conversations taking place of the shores of the Red Sea as the last of the Israelites climbed to a safe perch on the shore. Still looking at miraculous walls of water on both sides and a sky filled with fire their eyes settled only on the racing chariots of their former captors. "They're going to reach us and take us back to bondage!" "Help! We're no match for their power and might!" But just when the screams and fright grew to a new level, the Lord had a fresh command. Read Exodus 14: 26-31. What did God command Moses to do in verse 26 and what was the result?

_____

_____

_____

In one simple move of Moses' hands, the sea crushed the Israelites' opponents. I wonder if we realize the power of our hands. We've long been taught that struggles begin in our minds, and that's true—but they play out through our hands.

Today, our hands reach for healthy and life-giving food. Our hands grasp one another to join in mounted prayer. Our hands create beauty and present gifts of kindness. Like Moses, our hands smother the lies of darkness and bring forth the power of light.

Jesus, You are the light of the world. Let our lives reflect Your stunning radiance. Amen.

—— DAY 6: REFLECTION AND APPLICATION

Lord God, the power of your presence is no match for fear. No weapon meant for destruction will harm me.

We started the week by learning the word exodus means "get out of my way." This is a chant to remember, especially when we feel overcome by fear or stale with doubt. I find the more I say something, the more I believe it, and the more I believe it the more I live it. One of the most comforting yet powerful psalms is Psalm 23. Known for the gentleness of the Shepherd, it's also a hammer on the head of the enemy. Because this psalm is so well-known and easy to remember, let's add commentary to the beloved words of victory and hope.

Psalm 23

The Lord is my shepherd, I lack nothing. *I don't need to fill my life with things that are shallow...especially food.*

He makes me lie down in green pastures, He leads me beside quiet waters. *I have rest in Him and I'm not compelled to reach for substitutes.*

He refreshes my soul. He guides me along the right paths for his name's sake. *He fills me and completes me. He leads me in the perfect way so I can glorify His name.*

Even though I walk through the darkest valley, I fear no evil for You are with me; Your rod and Your staff, they comfort me. *No matter what happens or how bad things look, nothing is as real as Your presence. You protect and assure me in supernatural ways.*

You prepare a table before me in the presence of my enemies. You anoint my head with oil; my cup overflows. *Right in front of the enemy who threatens me, You prepare a calm meal for the two of us. You have given me purpose and the ability to live it out.*

Surely Your goodness and love will follow me all the days of my life, and I will dwell in the house of the Lord forever. *Healing and hope are mine forever. Nothing can ever separate me from my Lord.*

Dearest Savior, this psalm is mine to cherish forever. Amen.

—— DAY 7: REFLECTION AND APPLICATION

Father, this day I sing a new song to You: a song of love, praise, and victory. Amen.

Throughout the Bible after a stunning victory or even in times of confusion or apparent defeat, songs were a part of the landscape. After the waters closed in on the Egyptians in the book of Exodus, Moses and his sister Miriam led the Israelites in a song. The song was a description of what they'd just lived through that highlighted the majesty and power of God. As they sang of how the "horse and driver" were hurled into the sea—they rested upon a few choruses that we should sing...even today. Hum these verses today or write them in your journal.

◊   The Lord is my strength and my defense; He has become my salvation. (Exodus 15:2)

◊   The Lord is a warrior; the Lord is His name. (vs. 3)

◊   Your right hand, Lord, was majestic in power. Your right hand, Lord, shattered the enemy. (vs. 6)

◊   Who among the gods is like You, Lord? Who is like You—majestic in holiness, awesome in glory, working wonders? (vs. 11)

◊   In Your unfailing love You will lead the people You have redeemed. In Your strength You will guide them to Your holy dwelling. (vs. 13)

Father, we sing of your greatness from the core of who we are. There is none like You. Amen.

WEEK THREE: BATTLE SCARS

SCRIPTURE MEMORY VERSE
From now on let no one cause me trouble, for I bear on my body the marks of Jesus.
Galatians 6: 17

I have several scars on my body I'm quite proud of. Three cesareans, an appendectomy, skin cancer removal, biopsies, and too many skinned knees and cuts to count. Research shows the tissue under a scar heals stronger than the tissue before the blow. The circulation and health of the tissue is better than it was before the injury. This reminds us that what we see isn't always the true picture. When I look in the mirror, I may see a scar—but underneath is the healthy tissue of a healed wound.

Any one who lives *Beyond Free* has endured battles that inflict scars. I've never met a free person who hasn't experienced a few rounds with frustration or defeat. Thankfully, the scars are not the point, while the obedience leading to freedom is.

Most of us want to live an obedient life when it comes to our relationship with the Lord. The problem occurs when challenges deliver blows to our faith. Sometimes temptation pulls harder than grace, and we fall to the strike of the enemy. But what if we chose a better way? What if obedience was our ally instead of a wistful foe that lurks, waiting to make things difficult?

Author Beth Moore says, "Obedience is the mark of authentic surrender to God's authority in any matter."[1] *Living Beyond Free* requires this authentic surrender. There's simply no other way. But surrender isn't giving up...it's giving over. We give over what hasn't worked in the past. We give over the belief that our way is the right way and God's way is an option. We give over the cycles of defeat that make us want to quit trying.

This week we'll be learning about the ugly nature of our enemy. He'll do everything he can to discourage us, defeat us, and leave us in a heap on the side of the spiritual road. Thankfully, battle scars are proof of winning a well-fought fight. Our freedom quest is a stunning story of resolve versus resignation, courage versus retreat, and truth versus deceit. As we study our enemy and the overpowering hand of God, we move closer to our victory chant and the calm assurance that we are free! If we remain true to obeying his voice and his call, we can't fail. I believe obedience is the key to maturity, and maturity is the key to living *Beyond Free*.

—— DAY 1: YOUR SCHEMATIC PLAN

Lord Jesus, You have a plan for my life, and I joyfully surrender to it. Amen.

Before electricians wire a building they study the building's schematic. This plan typically looks like a diagram or flow chart that shows how the various parts of the building work, interact, or function. Our brains also function schematically. Every experience we have—every memory or connection to sights, smells, or sounds—interfaces with what we know as we try to make a connection. Schematic paths light up across our brains as we learn new things or come to new understanding. So, what does that have to do with our pursuit of freedom? Everything.

Just as God has a plan for our lives, the enemy has a schematic drawn up too. He's studied our tendencies, reactions, likes, dislikes, experiences, and dreams. The Apostle Paul speaks of schematics when he warns us about the way the enemy plots.

Please read Ephesians 6:11. What word did Paul use to describe the devil's action and what did he tell us to do?

_____

_____

Now turn to 2 Corinthians 2:11. Please write this verse below.

_____

_____

Instead of focusing on the armor God tells us to put on, we're going to look at this from another angle. We're going to look at the schemes. Paul says "don't be unaware" of them, and he warned the Ephesians to stand firmly.

If we were to dissect the schematic the enemy has drawn for us, there'd be three core tenants he attacks:

1. **Identity:** Who God has created you to be
2. **Purpose:** What God has created you to do
3. **Provision:** How you acknowledge who God has created you to be and accomplish what He has called you to do

It's important to note that God and Satan are not equal when it comes to schematics. God is all-powerful and all-knowing—Satan is not. The devil typically recycles the same techniques depending on our unique reaction to them. After he has collected data by watching our behaviors and tendencies, the schematic is set. He then uses lies, deceit, accusations, and distractions to keep us running in circles.

From the list above, which do you tend to struggle more from: identity, purpose, or provision? Why? Can you think of some life events that have influenced your schematic?

_____

_____

_____

From the time we're born till we take our last breath, our lives are influenced, challenged, and impacted by what we experience and how we create meaning from those experiences. When I was a young girl, my grandma would make delicious breakfasts. She'd fire up the griddle and cook crisp bacon, then she'd pour the batter for hot cakes that sizzled in the grease until perfectly crisp. We'd cover them in honey from a little ceramic bee she kept the honey in. Even though I don't eat hotcakes like that anymore, I have her ceramic bee on my shelf, and just the scent of honey brings a rush of emotions and mental connections. This is a nice connection that played into my schematic for years to come. My grandma's house was a place of normalcy and helped shape my identity. It was a refuge in my chaotic and violent world as a child.

Other types of schematic connections in our lives are not so nice. Bullying, abuse, neglect, loneliness, or the strange sense you don't fit in—all add to the schematic the enemy uses to steer us away from the goodness of the Lord. In his book When the Enemy Strikes, Dr. Charles Stanley explains the enemy's objective:[2]

- To draw us away from God. That's always the enemy's ultimate objective.
- To thwart God's purpose and plan for our lives. The enemy seeks to get us off track and out of the will of God.
- To deny God the glory, honor, and praise due Him as we live godly lives of faith and trust.
- To destroy us—literally and eternally.

Whew...heavy stuff! But friends, ignorance is not bliss. Understanding where the real fight for freedom takes place and whom we're fighting sets us up to win. Let's follow the apostle Paul's schematic and see how both the Lord and the enemy worked within.

Please turn to Philippians 3:4-6. How did Paul describe himself?

_____

_____

_____

That's a strong resume, and I sense his accomplishments and achievements are part of his prideful schematic. Dr. Stanley explains a "point of access" in which the enemy pushes in. For Paul, it seems his academic prowess and "righteous" ability to following all the rules was a perfect place for the enemy to camp.

Now turn to Acts 8:1-3. What type of scheme did the enemy use in Paul's life, based on what you know about his background?

_____

_____

_____

We tend to underestimate the terror Paul brought to the early church. He was literally dragging people who confessed Jesus into prison. Pregnant women, women with babies, men who were the sole provider of a family—he was ruthless. The enemy's entry point in Paul's schematic was pride.

Now turn to Acts 9:1-19. What did the Lord do to change the course of Paul's life?

_____

_____

I'm struck by the way Ananias lived. He knew Paul's reputation and the reason he was on his way to Damascus, yet Ananias followed a vision the Lord gave him about Paul's future. That's faith! His obedience led to the commissioning of one of the most dynamic and powerful apostles. If it weren't for Paul, we wouldn't have much of the New Testament.

During three blind days the Holy Spirit changed Paul's schematic, and the Spirit still can change ours. As we close out today, reflect on some points of entry in your life. Are there areas of doubt and defeat the enemy wrote across a diagram with your name on top? It may look like times you were betrayed or offended, times you chose the world rather than Jesus, or times you felt blind-sided by confusion

or fear. Ask the Holy Spirit to reveal these areas to you today.
Points of entry:

» _____
» _____
» _____
» _____

Now pray this prayer out loud with me.

Lord Jesus, I'm in awe of the intricate way You know me. I give all the events and memories in my life to You—the author and perfecter of my faith. There isn't one point of entry or one path on the schematic of my life that isn't touched by You. You have the ultimate plan, and nothing can touch it that won't be used for my ultimate good. Give me the courage to fight the battles I'm meant to fight and release the things that cause me to struggle. In Your mighty name I pray. Amen.

—— DAY 2: WHO IS THIS RIVAL?

Some people think the devil is a cartoonish guy dressed in a red suit, and others wink at him, acknowledging he exists but remaining unaware of his threats. It's certainly not healthy to over-study the enemy (we want to focus on Jesus and enjoy his abundance), but refusing to study him yields consequences that leave us in the dark.

I've loved Jesus for over thirty-seven years and experienced my share of battles, but this past year has shown me a side of the enemy I wasn't aware of. Before I share my experience, let's put some fences around what we know about the enemy and how Jesus described him.

Turn to the following scriptures and write a word or two to describe what the enemy is called.

John 8:44: _____
John 10:10: _____
Revelation 12:10: _____
2 Corinthians 11:3: _____
1 Peter 5: 8: _____

In addition to these descriptors Paul says, "For our struggle is not against flesh and blood, but against the rulers, against the authorities, against the powers of this dark world and against the spiritual forces of evil in the heavenly realms" (Ephesians 6:12).

It's enough to make our hair stand on end. But rest assured, the power of Jesus in you dismantles the enemy's power with a mere glance of authority. Let's learn more about that authority.

Defeating a foe becomes easy when you learn his strategy of attack. Satan is not creative. He uses a variation of the same tactics on every single human. The success he has creating chaos depends on our reaction to the way he attacks. Here are his four strategies:

- He attacks our **minds** through thoughts, ideas, suggestions, or excuses.
- He attacks our **mouths** as we speak what's been on our minds.
- He attacks our hearts to confuse our allegiance to God and commitment to His ways.
- He attacks our **bodies**, making it difficult to live out his promises and the dreams we have for this life.

The key is—depending on our schema (life experiences and how we make sense of them) and our neediness or wounds—he sends attacks designed to appeal to us. For instance, many people might not give a table full of food a glance, but food screams to a compulsive eater all night. Heaping plates, repeated trips to the table, and shoveling in leftovers when no one is looking all reflect a system based on Satan's lies. First, he sends messages and suggestions about food. We feel as though we need it, we deserve it, we can't resist it, it's our body, and we'll do whatever we want to with it. Soon, if we continually entertain these thoughts and allow them to control us, our bodies are enslaved to the strategy that began in our minds.

Read 1 Peter 1:13-16. How can we keep our minds safe?

_____

_____

_____

Now turn to Colossians 3:2-10. What did Paul instruct in these verses?

_____

_____

If you've been a Christian for a while, these concepts are not new to you, but why are they hard to live by? They're hard because just as the Lord's mercies are new every morning, the enemy's schemes are too. Just when we overcome one thing, he introduces another. Thankfully, the more we mature, the more we're alert to his stink.

I recently learned something new about the enemy that I'll never forget. I run a ministry in Uganda called The Vine and was preparing to leave the next day for a trip I anticipated would be hard. I prayed for a year that God would reveal things to me about my executive director and co-founder. He was like a son to me, but some things weren't adding up. I knew it'd be a difficult trip of discovery.

The day before I left my phone began acting up, so I popped into the phone store to get it checked. After several rounds of assistance by the salesman, he went into a back room and came back with a sticky note. It had the name of my email carrier on it, and he said to call that company, and it would assist me quickly in fixing the problem. I called the minute I got in the car and instantly the kindest, most thoughtful salesman began to help with my problem. He realized he couldn't fully help without my being on my laptop screen, so he offered to wait till I made the quick drive home. Once home, we opened up the screen and he accessed it to see what the problem was. (This is how most companies assist in repairs today.) He asked just the right questions regarding my history and needs. "Do I send a lot of international e-mails?" "Yes." "Wow, your email drive is tainted with hundreds of corrupt messages," he said sympathetically, as I watched a list of corrupt files pass over my laptop screen. After a few minutes he offered a way, the only way, for this to get fixed—a fee paid on-line to my e-mail carrier's company.

Every time I thought the call was strange, I reminded myself the phone store man gave me his number, so surely it was fine. Plus, I needed this to work since I was leaving for Africa the next day. What made it worse was he truly was the nicest guy, asking me questions about our Ugandan orphans and the work we do. At one point he even created a happy face on the screen. So sweet.

Before I paid for the service, I began to shake, and the Lord's discernment came over me. I told him I thought this was a scam and instantly he began to wipe things off my laptop. Programs and files were disappearing before my eyes before I could shut the system off. I was so upset for two reasons. I had believed a lie, and I had trusted someone who boldly took advantage of that trust. Little did I know the Lord was setting me up for my weeks in Africa, where I needed to realize the depths of evil. Had I not experienced that before I went, I probably wouldn't have been alert to the devastating power of deception. Oh, and by the way, I marched right into the phone store the next day and reported that salesman.

Lord, often I miss the stench of deception because it's hard to believe it's real or that bad. Show me areas I've tolerated or been tricked, and expose anything that's been held by sin. Amen.

—— DAY 3: FROM TOEHOLDS TO STRONGHOLDS

Jesus, You are the way, the truth, and the life. Nothing comes close to the love I have for You. Amen.

When I fell in love with Jesus, I came to Him with a messed-up mind. Deep in the throes of anorexia and compulsive behaviors with food, I laid my messy life at his feet and sighed in relief. I'd never heard words like salvation or sanctification. If I had, I probably would have run for the hills. Instead, I called a college friend I knew was a Christian. I was shaking as I dialed her number, and after explaining to her that I'd fallen in love with Jesus, I told her my problem.

"I feel like there's a war in my head. I love Jesus so much but it's like there's a screaming match in my brain and I want it to stop."
She calmly said, "Gari, there is a war in your head, but you have the power to overcome it. Jesus is the commander—you have all his power and the right to tell anything that isn't from him to go!"

I'm forever grateful for this friend. In one quick conversation she assured me I wasn't crazy, I wasn't alone, and I had power to wield in the heavenlies. Friends, so do you.

Please read 2 Corinthians 10:3-5. What kind of weapons are we fighting with?

_____

_____

_____

Paul stated the weapons we fight with are so strong they have divine power and are able to demolish strongholds (vs. 4). Write these four words from verse 4 below: divine, power, demolish, and strongholds.

_____

Divine power demolishes strongholds.

Nothing is truer than this statement. The problem is we often don't recognize our own strongholds, and we're not sure of our divine power to fight them. Let's take a few moments to better understand.

The Bible speaks often of strongholds. Ironically, the word was originally used as a place of refuge with the Lord until the enemy barged his way into its meaning. In Psalm 9:9 King David says, "The Lord also will be a stronghold for the oppressed, A stronghold for those in trouble" (NASB). What a beautiful picture of resting in the stronghold of God.

Most of our connotations today regarding a stronghold have to do with things we struggle with, and that is what Paul alluded to in his writing to the Corinthians. This definition of stronghold is a recurring, compulsive thought pattern that produces skewed behavior. Fortunately, we don't dive into the deep end of a stronghold. It starts with putting our toes in, then our feet, and eventually we're neck-deep in the water.

Dr. Stanley says, "If Satan is capable of deceiving you, craftily manipulating you and seducing you to yield to temptation in one area of your life, he's going to come back again and again to that area. He has identified this as an area of weakness. This area of weakness in you, becomes a stronghold for him."[3] So how do we deal with toeholds before they become strongholds? What is the secret to success?

On Day One we talked about the schematic the enemy has for our life based on our experiences and behaviors. We also explored the points of entry he has gained through our pain, confusion, or poor choices. For all of us, there's a point of entry moment that can define the outcome of many moments to come. It's a moment we can stand up to deceit—changing the course of our future. Point of entry (POE) moments either give the devil access or give God power. In these moments we either grow or slow the purposes of the Holy Spirit in our lives. The Bible is full of people who made wrong choices—inviting jealousy, greed, torment, and discouragement into their lives. But it's also full of those who got it right. At critical junctures they refused to give the devil a chance. Let's follow Daniel through several POE moments and apply this wisdom to our own.

Turn to Daniel 1:8-9. What action did Daniel take that set him apart?

_____

_____

Although no one would blame Daniel for feeling bad (he was taken from his home, ripped from his culture, and placed in a heathen palace to serve a corrupt king), at a critical moment he made up his mind to behave in a godly manner. Instead of inviting self-pity or helplessness, he set himself apart by the way he handled food. Instead of trouble, this brought favor from the very people who captured him. Here's our first POE moment action: **Make up your mind.**

It only takes three seconds to make a good choice. Count it: one, two, three. In the time a thought strikes to grab food, eat too much, or sneak something no one will see—in three quick seconds—we can walk away. Make up your mind this minute you won't choose food over obedience.

In his second year in Babylon there was another POE moment. Read Daniel 2:10-18. What precise actions did Daniel take to overrun fear and defeat?

_____

_____

_____

Instead of wringing his hands in defeat, he believed he could interpret the dream, even though he probably didn't know how. Most scholars think he was only about 17 years old when he made this bold claim. He also ran to ask his friends to pray for him before attempting what he'd never done. Another moment to note: instead of isolating and hiding in his task, he invited those he trusted to pray. Our second POE moment action: **Believe you can be successful even if you're not sure how. Ask for the help of those you trust. Strength rises on the backs of those who believe.**

How does being in a First Place group encourage you to believe you can be successful? Is there someone you need to ask to pray for you? (I'm not talking about token prayer, but rather, powerful, life-changing prayer that believes for great things.)

_____

_____

_____

Now turn to Daniel 6:1-10. Verse 10 is a paramount POE moment in the life of Daniel. What did he boldly do despite the king's verdict?

_____

_____

This leads us to our third POE moment action: **Stay on your knees no matter who is watching. When the enemy shuts doors, fling the windows open wide.**

Finally, read vs. 16-28. Note the impact Daniel's faith had on the king.

_____

_____

The fourth POE moment action: **Tested faith brings about assurance—not only in the one tested, but in those who watch the test.**

Which one of Daniel's point of entry moments reminds you of where you are in your life today? How can you respond as he did to your challenges?

_____

_____

_____

Lord, there are so many moments in a day. Teach me to foresee the moments that change my history, so I can respond as You would want me to respond. Amen.

—— DAY 4: BATTLE OF THE HORNS

Holy Spirit, Your Word is full of life. Thank You for both the deep and simple ways You use it to change me. Forever Yours…amen.

I looked out over the cornfields surrounding the Ugandan church I was to speak in that night. The half-built walls of brick weren't high enough to make a roof, but the crowd was gathering—not for a fancy church or slick production, but for the truth of God's Word and praise that ascended straight to the pulse of God. Before I spoke, the pastor took the dented microphone and began to preach from the words of the prophet Zechariah:

> "Then I looked up, and there before me were four horns. I asked the angel who was speaking to me, 'What are these?' He answered me, 'These are the horns that scattered Judah, Israel and Jerusalem.' Then the Lord showed me four craftsmen. I asked, 'What are these coming to do?' He answered, 'These are the horns that scattered Judah so that no one could raise their head, but the craftsmen have come to terrify them and throw down these horns of the nations who lifted up their horns against the land of Judah to scatter its people.'" (Zechariah 1:18-21)

I sat there, mesmerized by his cadence and authority. What were these horns he spoke of? I knew they had meaning but I'd never heard one single message about horns. He ended by quoting Psalm 75:10. Turn to this scripture and describe what God does to the horns.

_____

_____

_____

The NIV translation says God will cut off the horns of the wicked and lift the horns of the righteous.

This week we've studied the enemy's use of schematics and the way he wrangles sin into strongholds. Today, it's all about the horns. Day Three we spent time with Daniel observing how he handled point of entry moments that clearly defined his life. The enemy stands at those moments and brags he has defeated us. What a joy it is to blindside him with obedience. We are going to join Daniel again today as he interprets a strange vision that involves...you guessed it... horns.

Please read Daniel 7:1-8. What do we read in verse 8 about horns?

_____

_____

_____

Although this scripture is a confusing vision describing the political climate of Daniel's times (each animal represents Babylon, Persia, Greece, and Rome), our focus is the horns of the last beast in the vision.

What word describes how the horn is speaking (vs. 8)?

_____

Now let's read Daniel 7: 9-14. What's the most stunning thing you see in these verses?

_____

_____

What happens to the boastful horn (vs. 11)?

_____

_____

In these verses Daniel sees the Son of Man (Jesus) presented to the Ancient of Days (the Father). Describe what was given to Jesus by the Father (vs. 14).

_____

_____

We don't understand everything about this vision (neither did Daniel—as the vision was for the future to come) but some things are perfectly clear. The enemy is a boasting, arrogant voice before God. In these scriptures that voice comes from the horn of a beast. Typically, animals fight with their horns. They charge and lock horns to see who will overpower the other. In this stunning scene of the Son being presented to his Father, the nagging voice of arrogance tried to drown out worship for the Messiah King.

It's the same for us today. The enemy's goal is to lock horns with us and drown out our worship. How critical it is to realize the enemy's voice is destroyed as all power, authority and glory is given to Jesus by the Father.

Carole Lewis, one of the original members of First Place for Health and its national director emeritus says, "The devil's voice is mean, but the Holy Spirit's voice is kind." This is important to remember when we're sorting through what type of voices we listen to. In Daniel's vison it was the horn of a monster bragging arrogantly in the presence of God. This voice was so obnoxious it distracted Daniel from the beauty of the Father and Son until the voice was destroyed.

What does that voice look or sound like to you? For me, it's a megaphone or relentless nagging voice that replays the same discouraging messages. Take a few moments to draw or describe what the enemy sounds like.

_____

_____

Let's close today by looking at two additional references to horns. Read Psalm 89:24 then Luke 1:69. In Psalm 89 the word horn symbolizes strength and in Luke it means strong king. How do these horns outmatch the bragging arrogance of the enemy?

_____

_____

Father, the audacity of the enemy to boast in the presence of Your Son is unthinkable. Thank You that all power and authority is Yours forever. Amen.

—— DAY 5: THE VOICE

Lord, life can get pretty overwhelming at times. Show me how to become stronger by empowering others. In Jesus' name, amen.

The number one question I'm asked as a Bible teacher is, "How do you know the voice of God? How do you know he's speaking?" Some call God's voice "small and still," but I've always struggled with that. Instead, I think it is bold, assuring, and active. Because Jesus is God in the flesh, it's helpful to listen to the rhythm of what He says and how He says it. The more we learn to recognize His voice, the less likely we are to be deceived by Satan's. To begin, let's look at four different titles Jesus gave Himself and the unique voice that permeates each.

Turn to John 10:1-16. What title did Jesus give Himself?

_____

_____

I've read these verses hundreds of times, but I'm still amazed by their power. Before calling Himself "the good shepherd," Jesus called Himself "the gate" (vs. 7). What do you think He meant?

_____

_____

In a Messianic tone Jesus was referring to the fact He is the only way into God's Kingdom. There is absolutely no exception. In verse 10 He decisively called the enemy a thief. He boldly stated the difference between both their purposes. List the differences below:

Jesus's purpose: _____

The thief's purpose: _____

This is important because we often get confused. The thief thinks only of ruining everything good. Let's make this personal. Here's a list of things the enemy often tries to steal, kill, and destroy. Mark any you've experienced.

- o   You celebrate several consecutive days of discipline with food only to over eat and spiral into a worse cycle.
- o   You want to feel happy for those who look good, lose weight, and establish new habits—but all you feel is envy and frustration.

- o   The minute you wake up your mind is already reciting negative statements about who you are and the day you'll experience.
- o   You want to live differently, but the desire soon wanes in the face of food you crave. You beat yourself up for not having more self-control.
- o   You're snippy and critical when things don't go your way. The smallest thing can ruin an otherwise fine day.

Jesus was explaining that the thief's ways are cunning. He usually doesn't come right out and kill us, but he does kill our joy, peace, satisfaction, and hope.

What are some characteristics you note about the good shepherd in verses 11-15?

_____

_____

Unlike the large sheep farms we see today, in Jesus's day a shepherd cared for flocks that averaged forty sheep. The shepherds walked and spent all day and night with the sheep. They didn't have much of a social life outside of the sheep, and they were even known to name each sheep with a special name.

The key to the shepherd's commitment comes in verse 15. What did Jesus say about his life?

_____

_____

_____

Jesus said he lays down his life for the sheep, and I wonder, is there anything you'd lay down your life for? Most of us would say our spouse and children. That's usually a given. But a few years ago I had to think very carefully about this statement. I taught elementary school for many years, and our school was ten minutes from the first publicized school shooting at Columbine High School. As a matter of fact, our playground overlooked a cemetery that eventually housed the crosses marking the memorials for all the children who lost their lives that day.

On back-to-school night the following year I stood in front of a room full of parents and told them I'd lay down my life for their kids. In the event of a school shooting, I knew I was the only protection and "parent" their children had. This was a particularly hard sacrifice because my own small children were in the same building a few class-rooms away. Being with someone else's children meant I couldn't be with my own.

A good shepherd does not value his own life as much as he values the lives of those he cares for and protects. Jesus didn't put conditions on his sacrificial mandate—it was for all sheep, even those who stray or aren't thankful for the sacrifice.

In contrast, the prophet Ezekiel described a bad shepherd. Turn to Ezekiel 34:1-6. What are some of the flaws of a bad shepherd?

_____

_____

This passage is not only a warning to anyone who leads a ministry or congregation, but also a description of the way the enemy destroys. Let's compare the leadership styles of the good and bad shepherds.

Bad Shepherd: (our enemy)
- Cares only for himself
- Rules with force and cruelty
- Abandons and scatters the sheep
- Tricks and deceives the sheep with no remorse

Good Shepherd: (our Savior)
- Feeds and nourishes the flock
- Rules with love
- Gathers and protects the sheep
- Gives his life to shield those He loves

Given the characteristics above, can you detect a voice in your life that's not tender, nourishing, or protective?

_____

_____

Let's close today with the stunning words of Revelation 7:17. Write a short prayer of thanks to God for His beautiful promise.

_____

_____

My Shepherd, Your voice is all I hear. Thank You for your relentless pursuit. Amen.

—— DAY 6: REFLECTION AND APPLICATION

Dearest Lord, I thank You for my scars as they prove I was brave enough to battle. Amen

On Day Three we defined the word stronghold as most people see it today: "a recurring, compulsive thought pattern that produces skewed behavior." But before the word held a negative affiliation, it was used to describe the affection and protection of God. David was particularly fond of the word and used it many times in the Psalms he wrote. Let's spend some time today reflecting on the original use of this word.

> *"But as for me, I shall sing of Your strength;*
> *Yes, I shall joyfully sing of Your lovingkindness in the morning,*
> *For You have been* **my stronghold**
> *And a refuge in the day of my distress.*
> *O my strength, I will sing praises to You,*
> *For God is* **my stronghold**, *the God who shows me lovingkindness."*
> *Psalm 59:16-17 (NASB)*

David penned this psalm as he was lamenting defeat in battle and asking God for help. The stronghold represented a place people went for refuge to hide from danger, and David knew God was the stronghold of his life. He also knew God was the one who understood his worry and his moods. Goodness knows, our worry and moods could use a safe stronghold!

> *"When my anxious thoughts multiply within me,*
> *Your consolations delight my soul.*
> *But the Lord has been my stronghold,*
> *And my God the rock of my refuge."*
> *Psalm 94:19, 22 (NASB)*

Jesus, You are my stronghold, my refuge, and the place I hide. Amen.

—— DAY 7: REFLECTION AND APPLICATION

Lord, I want to understand who I really am, so I can be all I am meant to be. Please teach me today. Amen.

Reflect on the three words we considered on Day One.

- » **Identity:** Who God has created you to be
- » **Purpose:** What God has created you to do
- » **Provision:** How you will acknowledge what God has created you to be and accomplish what He has called you to do

If we aren't sure of our identity, our purpose is tainted; and if we aren't convinced of our purpose, we don't trust for provision. Talk to you First Place for Health group or prayer partner about which area you tend to struggle with the most. Commit that area to prayer for the upcoming week.

Sweet Savior, my identity is in You. You give my life meaning and purpose. Amen.

Notes:

1. Beth Moore, "Breaking Free: A 5-Day Reading Plan." https://www.bible.com/reading-plans/3830-breaking-free/day/4.

2. Charles Stanley, When the Enemy Strikes (Nashville: Thomas Nelson Publishers, 2004), 116.

3. Ibid, p. 77.

WEEK FOUR: BREAKING GENERATIONAL CYLES

SCRIPTURE MEMORY VERSE

"See, the former things have taken place, and new things I declare; before they spring into being I announce them to you."
Isaiah 42: 9

This week's lessons have me in tears. Good tears...steeped in awe and praise. If you have broken free from a past filled with pain, you know what I mean. From the time I was a child, generational curses held my parents, grandparents, and their parents in a chokehold of shame. Repeating the same cycles of defeat, we succumbed to the terror of addiction, compulsion, alcoholism, adultery, manipulation, and abuse. But no more! The day I said yes to Jesus was the day I began to pursue freedom. The power of God in Christ is no match for the chains of slavery. But sadly, many believers are wrapped in chains they themselves did not place there. The chains of parents, grandparents, teachers, coaches, churches, spouses, friends, and even certain business establishments can become our chains if we're not careful.

In his book *Wild at Heart* John Eldredge speaks about the wounds we experience in life—the places of shame, the hurt, and the scars from an imperfect past. He says God is fiercely committed to us and to the restoration of our hearts, but a wound that goes unacknowledged and unwept is a wound that won't change. [1] "A wound you've embraced is a wound that cannot heal. A wound you think you deserved is a wound that cannot heal."[2]

I spent years embracing wounds that were passed down to me without my understanding. How beautiful it is to realize we're not bound by the sin or problems of those who've gone before us. We don't blame people or sit in morbid reflection of what's transpired—instead, we rise up in strength as we allow the Lord to cleanse our hearts and set us free.

—— DAY 1: THE FIRST STEP

Jesus, You broke every curse when You became a curse on the cross. We worship You and thank You for your sacrifice. Amen.

No one can argue that our families and those who have influenced our past hold a stake in helping to form who we have become. For some of us that's a beautiful gift. If you had wonderful parents and a childhood filled with support, you were given a valuable head start in the race of life. For the rest of us, it may feel as though we have been trying to run with heavy weights strapped to our ankles.

To be clear, after I came to faith in Christ, I never wanted to look back—and certainly don't endorse a mindset that overanalyzes or places blame on people or past events. The Bible is a redemptive book of new chances and new design. The issue for me was I refused to consider where I'd been. I thought if I didn't acknowledge my past, perhaps it might not impact my future. That's a narrow way of thinking that hinders growth. True maturity is being able to look at our past without getting stuck there.

Read 2 Corinthians 5: 17. What does God say about our old creation?

_____

_____

_____

The Life Application Bible Commentary says, "Christians are brand new people on the inside. The Holy Spirit gives them new life, and they are not the same any more. We are not reformed, rehabilitated, or reeducated—we are new creations, living in vital union with Christ." This is fantastic news for every believer seeking to live a victorious life. The trouble is we often misunderstand that verse. It says the old has gone and the new is here—it does not say the old never happened and shouldn't be considered.

I didn't understand the power of generational cycles until I began to long to be free. I knew my behavior with food was compulsive, but I didn't know what to do about it. As I prayed, I remembered my grandfather. I adored him, but he struggled mightily with food. When we'd visit in the summer, throughout the night I'd hear the spoons rattling in the drawer as he'd get up several times to eat ice cream. When we woke, he'd already been to the donut shop and brought back freshly glazed donuts, several of which he ate in the car on the drive home. One summer he lost a lot of weight by not eating any solid food for months, but once he resumed normal intake, the weight came right back on. He eventually struggled with diabetes and died of a heart attack in the hallway of his home.

I soon recognized this as a generational cycle that needed to break if I wanted to truly be free from food bondage. The same is true for any type of bondage. Someone once said we're only as sick as our secrets. In the case of generational cycles, family secrets can snuff out the life of freedom God intends for us. Breaking generational patterns of destructive behavior changes not only our lives, but also the lives of our children, no matter how old they are. I've recognized four steps I believe are necessary in moving toward a new life and healing.

- **Acknowledge the past**, and name specific people and events that caused anguish, perpetuating a negative generational cycle.
- **Forgive your past** so it doesn't dictate your future.
- **Live like new**, as God recreates and regenerates what's been dead or damaged.
- **Seal your healing.** Mark it as a monument—a time you know you've en countered God.

For our purposes today, we're going to focus on acknowledging our past. In the world there are two forces at work—the flesh and the Spirit. Turn to Galatians 5:16-21. List out some of the behaviors of the flesh you see mentioned.

Has anyone impacted or harmed you by carrying out one or more of these behaviors? Explain.

Both my parents were alcoholics, and my grandfather had an eating disorder. Bobby's father and my father were both womanizers like their fathers before them. Sadly, the pain of all these destructive behaviors gravely impacted my childhood and life as a young adult. These generational cycles also made me ripe for compulsion and chaos.

Do you see a pattern of destructive behavior (sin) in your family that originated in the generations before you? (Think about your parents, grandparents, aunts, uncles, great-grandparents.)

How has this destructive pattern influenced the way you act or react? For instance, I struggled with great insecurity as my parents' alcoholism made them distant, abusive, and neglectful. As an adult I struggled to believe I really mattered to anyone. I've overcome this with years of believing the truth and the assurance that I matter to God. Reflect on your life. Do you see the effect of generational cycles?

_____

_____

_____

Most of the generational cycles of sin can be placed in three categories. Each of these categories has a behavior we adopt in reaction to the cycle of sin. See if you relate to any of the groups below.

» Growing up with compulsion, addiction, anger, which can lead to a sense of helplessness, victimization, low self-esteem.

» Growing up with manipulation and abuse of power or control, which can lead to people pleasing, lack of control, the need to overcontrol people out of fear.

» Growing up with sexual abuse, adultery, stealing, lying for gain, which can lead to a lack of trust, fear of betrayal, and difficulty letting people get close to you.

Let's see how the Bible describes the issue of generational sin. Turn to Ezekiel 18:14-20. What does verse 20 make clear?

_____

_____

_____

The child will not share the guilt of a parent. This is good news for those who've felt guilty for all kinds of unexplained things. It also offers comfort to parents who are afraid to pass down to their children what they reluctantly learned from theirs.

The idea of passing sins down generationally was a common theme for disciples in Jesus's day. Turn to John 9:1-6. What did Jesus teach his disciples through their misperception?

_____

_____

How refreshing to see hardships or things we've long struggled with instead as opportunities to see the works of God displayed! The first step to healing from generational cycles of sin is to acknowledge them. Once we do, we can begin to see the works of God displayed through them. Have you seen God work through a generational cycle of sin in your life or the life of someone you know? Acknowledge the cycle below.

Lord, I acknowledge the patterns of generational sin. I will neither ignore them or blame them. They display Your good works as I'm set free. Amen.

—— DAY 2: LETTING GO
Lord, I accept responsibility for any behavior that has created consequences in my life and determine to seek healthier practices. Amen.

One of the hardest things we face as believers is forgiving what's caused us harm. Because I ignored much of my childhood—pretending like it didn't hurt—I was unaware that unforgiveness was festering in my soul. Bouts of anxiety, insecurity, and a cranky self-image that saw things from a distorted point of view ran me around in circles.

One day Bobby and I were speaking to a large church audience. I was sharing a story from my childhood I typically made a joke of. It was Christmas morning, and my quadriplegic dad was brought to the house by the physical therapist he lived with after moving from our home shortly after his car accident. Mom started drinking early, and by mid-morning she beat my dad and pulled him out of his wheelchair. My little brother, sister, and I tried to pull him back into his

chair, but he was too heavy for us to lift. So, he lay in a strange position for hours on our hallway floor until the physical therapist came and got him. As dinner approached, I looked at the burnt turkey in the oven and poured three bowls of Cap'n Crunch for Christmas dinner.

Normally I laughed while telling this story, joking that I thought cereal was the only food group there was. But this day nothing seemed funny. It was as though the weight of a painful childhood finally broke like a stopped-up dam. After mucking around in the pain for a while I came upon some serious words of Jesus that alarmed me.

Turn to Matthew 6: 9-15. What do verses 14-15 teach about forgiveness?

_____

_____

_____

I love the "Our Father" prayer right above, but these sharp words from Jesus really cut through my soul. I'd been harboring unforgiveness toward both my parents for their cycles of sin, and what's worse, I never saw how it hindered my own growth.

Read Mark 11: 25-26. What did Jesus say we must do in order to enjoy the forgiveness He offers?

_____

_____

Forgiveness is not an option, it's a command. Thankfully, Jesus only commanded us to do things that greatly benefit us in the long run. He also understands how difficult forgiveness is, especially when the pain inflicted caused lasting damage.

Sometimes, a parent or person of influence may not even realize his or her behavior was detrimental. In the book of Genesis, Joseph's father Jacob showed great favoritism towards the sons of the wife he loved best, putting Joseph in great danger with his older brothers. Jacob's childhood was marred by a meddling mother who struggled with deception (Rebekah). She shoved that trait onto Jacob, who passed it down to his older sons...and so on.

The older brothers of Joseph probably had no idea they were perpetuating a generational curse. They were just doing what came naturally to them—lying, destroying, making poor decisions based on jealousy, and covering up.

Turn to Genesis 45:1-8. How did Joseph react when he acknowledged the pain he endured at his brothers' hands?

_____

_____

_____

What power do you see in Joseph's acknowledgment of pain?

_____

_____

_____

Joseph broke the power of his generational curse by forgiving his painful past, not ignoring or excusing it. How can you do the same? Is there someone or something you need to forgive?

_____

_____

_____

Don't let another minute pass with unforgiveness festering in your heat. Let's end today by praying this prayer together:

Dearest Father, I don't want to dwell on my past, but I also don't want to miss the chance to break off any chains that bind me to it. Holy Spirit, in these quiet moments of study, bring to remembrance anything You feel is important for me to acknowledge and forgive. Is there a person, or event You need me to note, so You can break the unhealthy hold or pattern its created in my behaviors? I ask You to show it to me now or in the weeks to come, as I can handle it. Whatever comes to mind, no matter how big or small, I will lay it at Your feet as You lovingly and decisively deal with it. The first step is to acknowledge it's there, and today I give You permission to reveal things I've forgotten or buried. The next step is to forgive the person who has hurt me. Free me from my anger or bitter resignation as You free my perpetrator's sin. Your ways are always tender and true. I ask You to break any generational cycles in my life and the life of my family. In Your mighty and matchless name, I pray. Amen.

—— DAY 3: IT'S A NEW DAY

Lord, how refreshing it is to realize I don't have to hang on to yesterday. I'm free to live a new tomorrow. Amen.

I love the before-and-after pictures in magazines. I look for the little details that together, add up to big change. It's amazing how the shift of a piece of furniture or a variation in color scheme can change the entire look of a room. The sweep of side bangs, a new lipstick color, or the belt around a baggy outfit leaves an entirely new impression. The same before-and-after effect is possible in our lives. I respect you too much to type out platitudes and trite sayings rather than truth. I was in the grip of generational sin for many years until I learned the Holy Spirit, in all His creative design, is famous for redecorating.

Days One and Two we talked about acknowledging and forgiving the damaging cycles passed down to us by former generations—now we get to the good stuff.

Turn to Ephesians 4:23-24. Why do you think Paul chose those words to describe the process of change?

_____

_____

_____

Paul said, "put on the new self...." He did not say to partially cover up, to hold it behind your back, or to keep living in the same old outfit. He said, "put on the new you." *Put it on!* Often, we're so stuck in who we were we can't see who can be.

I remember a time in my life I was stuck. Bobby's baseball career was at a halt, we had three small children, and I couldn't see a way forward no matter how hard I tried. I desperately wanted to write books but wasn't quite ready. I boldly called the editor of a sports magazine and asked him if he'd be interested in a story about the former New York Yankees shortstop. He reluctantly said to write it and send it in. Soon, I had a contract, which began an eight-year stint as a sports reporter. I allowed God to begin to re-make me, even though I was terrified, had low self-esteem, and wasn't even sure how to write. When the apostle Paul wrote to "put on the new self...," it came with the assurance that Jesus knows what your new self will be. The problem is after sinking to the weight of defeating cycles of sin, it's hard to picture ourselves in a new light.

Read the following scriptures and describe what happens as we put on new life.

Romans 6: 6-7_____

_____

2 Corinthians 5:17-18_____

_____

Psalm 19:7-9_____

_____

The next story has the power to change the trajectory of your life. I don't mean to oversell it, but I believe it's true. We can either stay stuck in the past or bland present—or believe for a glorious future ahead.

In an overlooked story in 2 Kings, the prophet Elisha teaches a stunning lesson to Joash, King of Israel. Elisha was sick and near his death when the king came to him for advice about a battle. Let's join the story there.

Read 2 Kings 13:14-21. What did Elisha ask the king to do in verse 17?

_____

_____

_____

It may seem strange that the prophet took the king's hands and shot an arrow out an open window, but there was great purpose in this act. The arrow was a symbol of battle and the east was the position of the enemy. As the arrow flew out the window, Elisha taught the king that the battle was already won for the Lord. This is important for us to remember. God always provides the arrows for us to position and conquer our enemy. He even places His hands on ours as we shoot. If we cower or never stand at the window to fight, we stay stuck in fear and resignation to a defeated stance.

The next part of the story is bizarre but profound. What did Elisha ask the king to do in verse 18?

_____

_____

_____

First, we saw the king shooting arrows out a window. Now he was asked to beat the ground with them. Imagine his confusion or pride in being asked to do something that seemed so silly! He reluctantly struck the ground but only three times as a token to the prophet. What did the prophet say to the king in verse 19?

_____

_____

Elisha was disappointed the King held back in his faith—either questioning what God instructed or already defeating it in unbelief. What if the King had taken handfuls of arrows and struck the ground for all he was worth? How would his life and battles have looked different? It's interesting that the final implication Elisha left on earth was,

"Believe for more than you can imagine, even if the way God uses to bring about the impossible seems confusing. Or worse...ridiculous!"

In that arrow moment, God was trying to redesign the belief system of the king. Some of us have been fighting the same battles, the same way, for a very long time. Perhaps it's time for you to take your arrows of desire, hope, good intent, dreams, and new action...and strike the floor with wild abandon. If we do the striking, He does the changing.

What one thing can we "take to the floor" today? How is this a step towards breaking generational cycles from the past?

_____

_____

_____

_____

_____

_____

Jesus, You redesign my life when I allow You full access. Like the arrows of Joash, I believe with complete abandon in the wonderful things You will do. Amen.

—— DAY 4: MARKING MOMENTS

Father, You bring me to life-changing moments. I promise to mark them, name them, and remember them. Amen.

In the flitting and flight of life, it's easy to fly past moments God has designed for us to pause. When we hear from God, understand something in a new way, sense He is stirring or teaching us in a profound way—these are moments we must mark as monuments. Monuments are the altars we build when we know life from this point on is different. We've encountered God. We're no longer the same.

This week we have talked about breaking generational cycles of destruction. After acknowledging the cycles, forgiving the perpetrator, and choosing to live a different way—there comes a point we mark the process of change with a monument. The Old Testament is full of them—altars erected to honor God and acknowledge His purpose and hope.

The first recorded monument appears in the life of Noah. Turn to Genesis 8:18-21.

How do you think Noah felt spiritually and emotionally when he finally stepped on dry ground? Why is building an altar in these moments significant?

_____

_____

_____

_____

After months on a dark, damp ark—floating on the uncertainty of what their future held next—Noah had only his faith to buoy him. I love that the first thing Noah and his family did was worship. Truthfully, I might have started to build a new home, scouted out the best place to plant crops, and begin a new life...but this is not what Noah did. The trauma of the flood led to a posture of worship. This is important. Some of us have been in a season of uncertainty, floating on unending waves of confusion or the drizzle of ambiguity. How exciting it is to remember that like Noah, dry shore is coming! And when we arrive there, we need to mark the moment with a monument of praise. Let's name this altar:

Monument #1:
The Lord leads to safe shores of new beginning.

Now turn to Genesis 12:6-7. What did God say to Abram in verse 7?

_____

_____

_____

_____

When Abram was 75 years old, he left the land of his father and went into the unknown. Certainly, he had the promise of God that he'd be blessed, but it's easy to forget God's promises when we travel long distances without sight of how we thought God would bless us.

The altar Abram built was in Shechem, which means "strength" in Hebrew. It's important to note that Abram wasn't yet where God promised, but he was still in a strong place. At times I'm so busy fretting I'm not where I want to be that I miss where I am. Shechem wasn't the final destination, but it was a strong one. It was a place God appeared to Abram—and ultimately, that's enough.

Monument #2:
We may not be where we want to be, but wherever God is, that's where we are.

Now let's look at Genesis 12:8 then 13: 3-4. Where did Abram settle and what did he do in this place?

_____

_____

_____

Scripture notes that Abram settled between Bethel on the west and Ai on the east. In this spot he built an altar and called upon the Lord. In his sojourning Abram found himself between two cities. Bethel means "house of God" and Ai means "heap of ruins." What a contrast, but what a monument. In this place—between the city of God and the city of ruin—he called on the name of the Lord. This is a powerful way to handle the pull towards deception and the tug of the world. When we're caught in between, we call on the name of our God.

Notice in Genesis 13:3-4 Abram ended up back in the same place. Fortunately, he'd already built a monument there. I believe that because he'd marked that monument as a time he'd heard from God, he was enabled to handle the next decision of his life with wisdom and a prophetic grace. At this symbolic place, he split from his relative Lot. Lot went on towards a place of grave evil, and Abram settled in his personal promised land.

Monument #3:
When camped between good and evil, call upon God.
Our monument leads to the land of promise and new life.

The final step in breaking generational cycles is marking the moments we see God move. Can you build a monument to God today? Is there something new or inspiring He is showing you? Is there something you want to mark as a monument—a place you know that God has touched and encountered?

_____

_____

_____

Oh Lord, I build an altar to You in praise. You have led me to this point in my life, and I thank You for all the experiences that have led me here. Amen.

—— DAY 5: CURSE BUSTERS

Dearest Lord, today we break the power of any verbal or nonverbal curse laid over our lives. We walk in Your new, redeeming power from this day forth. Amen.

As an elementary school teacher, I witnessed first-hand the damaging effect of teasing, harsh words, and bullying. Fragile little minds take the blows like a rubber stand-up clown. But soon, the smile fades and the effect of the blows overtakes any resilience to withstand. The truth is, "stick and stones may break our bones," but words will break our hearts.

Certain verbal curses may have been placed on your life knowingly or unknowingly. The words of a parent, teacher, coach, friend, pastor, or boss have the power to influence our self-image and distort the person God has created us to be. I can still remember certain phrases spoke over me that influenced my behavior as an adult. When mom was drunk, she said some awful things, and I vividly remember her saying she wished I'd disappear. She loved my brother and sister but wished I was gone. This set me up for decades of feeling as though I didn't matter to anyone. She often called me clumsy and withheld any type of compliment or encouragement. Thus, whenever I got around her, I was clumsy and struggled to be noticed. I became a people-pleaser with an insatiable need for strokes. Fortunately, our Jesus is a life speaker, and busts the curses spoken over us. Often, we're not aware that we're experiencing the effects of verbal curses.

Do any of these comments sound like things you've said about yourself recently?

- I'm a quitter.
- I have no self-control.
- I'm not smart enough to fulfill my dreams.
- I was born this way.
- God speaks to other people but not to me.
- I'm big boned and my body doesn't change.
- I'm _____(fill in the blank)
    - Quick-tempered
    - A pushover
    - Ugly and of no use
    - Out of control
    - An outcast, unlovable, unworthy

If you've answered yes to a few of these, chances are you're feeling the effects of a verbal curse. The whole notion of a "curse" can be confusing because we rarely use this language. It brings to mind witchcraft or Halloween games—not something we may struggle with on a daily basis. A curse is an utterance intended to harm or bring punishment on someone or something. It's also an offensive word or phrase used to express anger or annoyance. Even our term *curse word* is a reference to words spoken that are alarming, offensive, and rude and uttered out of the flesh not the Spirit.

We've spent this week looking at generational cycles and the steps to overcoming their effects. Today we'll study the last thing we need in our toolbox as we overcome the sting of verbal curses—the power to overcome the effect of someone else's tongue.

Turn to James 3:1-12. How does James describe the power of the tongue?

_____

_____

_____

Clearly, the tongue and how it's used are a big deal. James compares the damage the tongue can do to a raging fire. Satan uses the tongue to divide, confuse, and put down people, thus invoking all kinds of curses that seep into the crevices of the soul.

The problem is we often don't know how to detect Satan's curses. According to one commentary, here's a way to tell. Speech motivated by Satan is full of jealousy, selfishness, earthly concerns and desires, disorder, evil, *harsh criticism*. Speech motivated by God's wisdom is full of mercy, love for others, courtesy, peace, sincerity, gentleness, goodness, and *straightforward truth wrapped in love*.[3] The way we break the power of a generational verbal curse is by recognizing where it's come from—and refusing to give it one more minute of power over who we believe we are.

God often uses names in the Bible to break a former curse or rename someone for a better purpose. Let's look at some of the ways God reshaped the destiny of his people by changing their names.

Turn to Genesis 17:5. What was Abraham called before he was renamed?

_____

_____

God took Abram (high father) and changed him to Abraham (father of nations). His purpose in Abraham's life far outweighed how Abram had seen himself in his father's household.

Turn to Genesis 17:15. What was Sarah's name before God changed it?

_____

_____

God took Sarai's name (my princess) and changed it to Sarah (princess and mother of nations).

Finally, let's look at John 1:42. What was Peter's name originally?

_____

_____

Peter's former name Simon meant "God has heard." That's wonderful, but he was soon renamed "the rock." Before Jesus died on the cross, he occasionally called Peter by his old name Simon. Some scholars believe this is because at times, Peter was acting like his old self. But, as Peter led the New Testament church into power and purpose, his name was sure: Peter, the rock.
So why new names? Because new names are the way we overcome old identities and curses. A new name shows we're destined for a new mission. It's a way to live out the divine plan God has for us, and to be known as He sees us, not as the world cursed us.

Lord, rename me. I want to hear Your name for me ring from the chorus of my mind.

—— DAY 6: REFLECTION AND APPLICATION
Dearest Lord, what a pleasure it is to move beyond the cycles of pain passed from generations before me. I am free to live beyond their borders and control. Amen.

On Day Four we talked about the monuments (altars) marked in the Bible that represent a moment of remembrance. Often, the one who built the monument named it according to an attribute of God or something He had done.

If you could walk the rooms of my house, you'd see monuments in each room—reminders and markers representing an encounter I've had with God. In a beautiful soap dish by my kitchen sink I have a rock with a scripture from Nehemiah painted on it. It sits as a monument to the healing I've had with food and the freedom I walk in.

On my bedroom nightstand sits a framed scripture my son wrote during a terrible time in my marriage. It serves as a monument to the restored marriage we enjoy and the miraculous healing that took place in our relationship. Finally, on the desk in my office sits an antique glass bowl with rocks from Uganda. These serve as monuments marking the courage God has given me to do the impossible. Daily, these monument markers set my mind on the power of the God I serve.

Take time today to create a monument. You can use anything you'd like; the point is to set it somewhere strategic, so you'll continually see it and thank God for his power in your life. Consider sharing your monument with a family member or your First Place group.

Reflect on this from Exodus 17:15: "And Moses built an altar to the Lord and named it The Lord is My Banner."

Lord, I long to remember the mighty ways You work. I set aside altars of remembrance in my home to keep my eyes steadily on You. Amen.

—— DAY 7: REFLECTION AND APPLICATION

Father, I look forward to the new things You have planned. I won't cling to the past when the new awaits. I trust You with my "new." Amen.

Our memory verse for this week is, "See, the former things have taken place, and new things I declare; before they spring into being I announce them to you" (Isaiah 42:9). I love the fact that God declares new things over us before we're even aware. When we're fixated on the former things, we risk seeing the new things that God declares. A collection of "declares" is a declaration. As our founding fathers wrote the Declaration of Independence, we can write our own declaration and celebrate our freedom from anything that keeps us from God's call and purpose.

On the following lines, list some of your declarations and turn them into a prayer for the upcoming weeks we have together. Even if you're in the process of change and don't feel like you're there quite yet, supernatural power flows when we join God in declarations.

I Declare:

_____

_____

_____

_____

_____

_____

Father, we agree with what You declare and look forward to what springs forth from our faith. You are a God of new beginnings and hope. Amen.

Notes

1. I refer to this in my book Truly Fed: Finding Freedom from Disordered Eating (Kansas City: Beacon Hill Press, 2009).

2. John Eldredge, Wild at Heart (Nashville: Thomas Nelson, 2001), 106.

3. TLB Life Application Bible (Carol Stream, Ill.,: Tyndale House Publishers, 2012), 1921. Italics added.

WEEK FIVE: PLANTING NEW FIELDS

SCRIPTURE MEMORY VERSE
But the seed falling on good soil refers to someone who hears the word and understands it.
Matthew 13:23

There's something about a field that inspires me. Vast mounds of dirt and wild grass waiting to be tamed and to become fruitful and boast a meaningful crop that sustains and nourishes. This is the image God repeatedly uses to teach us about faith. Fields ready to be sown with fresh seed—promising new growth. It's a lofty idea, but how do we make it real in our day-to-day lives? What exactly does it mean to plant and harvest our cravings, habits, and behaviors? The Bible makes it clear that what we plant matters. The seeds we put into the soil of our lives will produce a crop. The question is: what kind of crop?

When I first began to get free, the principle of seed sowing was the catalyst to my change. I finally understood that gluttony was sin and that I was involved in a spiritual battle rather than a worldly fight. But at the end of the day, I still asked the simple questions. "What do I eat? How much should I eat? And how do I tame my craving for more?" These questions became the seed I planted.

When Jesus taught on seed and soil he was clear: the soil determines the yield. Soil is the condition of our heart. If our hearts are hard—the seed won't penetrate. If our hearts are shallow, the seed can't take root. And if our hearts are worried and negative, the seed is choked by thorns pretending to be nice.

Over the past few weeks we've looked at sin, the need for a personal exodus, battle scars, and problems passed down through the generation. This week it's all about the seeds—the daily choices and momentary decisions that change the landscape of our lives.

—— DAY 1: SEED POWER

Jesus, the seeds I sow in life matter. Help me to plant and nurture well. Amen.

When I taught third grade science, one of the units we covered was plant life. We'd take white Styrofoam cups and place just the right amount of soil in the bottom. Then, each student would lovingly place a seed in the soil and cover it. The cups sat on the windowsill, receiving a small amount of water each day, until miraculously... little stems and leaves appeared! We'd shout in amazement as the plants grew so tall they danced across our windows. To this day, I'm still amazed by the miracle. How do tiny hard seeds bring beauty and life?

If we could cut open a seed and watch its power in the soil, we'd see several interesting things happen. A seed has a protective coat around its shell that keeps it safe as it begins to grow. Inside the seed an embryo (baby plant) begins to stir. Through a burst of energy stored in the seed and a limited food supply—the plant takes shape. As the seed starts to grow, one part becomes the stem, and the other becomes the root. Both form at the same time. The stem grows up and the root grows down. Even when a seed is upside down in the soil, it will right itself. The seed's main goal is to reach the sunlight. The light and water will sustain it.

No wonder the Bible uses seeds, sowing, reaping, and harvest as principles for life. God protects us as we grow, and the Holy Spirit provides the energy and nourishment as we reach towards the Son and the living water. Even when we're upside down, we can right ourselves as God shows us how.

Please turn to Galatians 6:7-9. How does Paul explain the principle of seed sowing?

_____

_____

_____

_____

I credit Paul's words to the Galatians for cutting through my excuses—and laying my habits and behaviors bare. He's not messing around, and neither should we. Paul says two things: we shouldn't be deceived, and God cannot be mocked. He goes on to explain that when we sow seeds to please ourselves (our fleshly desires, appetites, and undisciplined whines and wants), we reap destruction. But when we sow to the Spirit, we reap life forever.

I used to think these verses were meant only for salvation—that perhaps Paul was specifically using them to bring people to eternal life—until I realized eternal life begins today. The moment we say yes to the love of the Lord Jesus, eternal life begins that day, that moment—not the day we die. This means as we sow seeds to the Spirit, we reap life every single day. But before we do a happy seed dance, let's look at the weight of what Paul has said. "Don't be deceived. ... God will not be mocked."

It's not that we want to play dumb and walk around mocking God. The trouble is we're often deceived and naively mock God with our behaviors or disbelief. I talk to countless women who tearfully tell me they've prayed for years to be free from bondage to food. Then I go out for a meal with them and they eat the richest thing on the menu and ask for dessert. There's a disconnection between desiring to change and the discipline it takes to get there.

One thing we need to make clear is God loves us regardless of our choices and behaviors. If we never lose a pound or exercise a step, God is crazy about us and loves us deeply with an unconditional love. But if our hearts cry out for freedom, and we truly want to change—we need to move beyond deception. Deception says, "I'm fine" or "I can't"—while mocking says, "God isn't concerned about my body" or "It's my body and I'll do with it what I want."

In my books *Truly Fed* and *Be Free*, I share the difference between sowing flesh seeds and spirit seeds. Circle any of the descriptions you relate to below.

Spirit Seeds

- Exposing food secrets.
- Understanding the truth about our bodies and habits
- Offering to God specific times we engage in damaging behaviors and choosing to change our actions and habits.
- Filling our minds with affirming phrases and scriptures rather than food

Flesh Seeds

- Hiding and lying about food.
- Denying that habits are destructive.
- Continuing behaviors that lead to guilt, shame, and secrecy.
- Reciting lies in our minds and remaining hopeless.

Sowing is a word used throughout the Bible to describe the action of scattering seeds, then nurturing and caring for their growth. We make choices every day regarding what we'll eat, how we'll eat, and how much or how little we'll eat. Our choices are the seeds we sow toward food. To a person not obsessed with eating, these choices are natural, simple, and unrestricted. To someone struggling with compulsive or habitual overeating, these choices are sown to the destruction of life.[1]

Please read Romans 8:6. How did Paul describe our minds when governed by the flesh and spirit?

Let's place our choices, attitudes, and habits with food in the context of sowing seeds. Honestly reflect and list which habits bring maturity and life and which bring destruction. Let's call the destructive patterns flesh seeds and the life-giving choices spirit seeds. Write them below.

Flesh Seeds:

_____

_____

_____

Spirit Seeds:

_____

_____

_____

Now turn to Romans 8:11-13. Please copy verse 13 below.

_____

_____

_____

You will live! Just like the little seed that grows in the darkness of the soil, your roots and branches form as you choose life. Soon, you'll be dancing on fertile field, ripe with new life.

Jesus, even little seeds bring forth Your plan for new life. In my moments of darkness, remind me I'm growing and stretching towards You. Amen.

—— DAY 2: HOW DO WE SOW?

Father, Your principle of sowing is simple yet deep. Show us how to comprehend the depth of what You are trying to teach. Amen.

When it comes to learning new things, I view my learning style as "show me" don't merely "tell me." Anyone can tell us what to do, but when someone shows us how, that's when we truly change. Today, I'm going to show you how to sow to the spirit when it comes to food.

Yesterday we considered Paul's instruction regarding sowing and reaping. There's no denying the truth—we reap what we sow. But just telling someone to sow good seeds is not enough. We need to understand how to sow and why. To begin, let's read the scripture we studied yesterday.

"Don't be misled; remember that you can't ignore God and get away with it: a man [or woman] will always reap just the kind of crop he sows! If he sows to please his own wrong desires, he will be planting seeds of evil and he will surely reap a harvest of spiritual decay and death; but if he plants the good things of the Spirit, he will reap the everlasting life the Spirit gives him." Galatians 6:7-9 (TLB Life Application Bible, parenthetical addition mine).

How are poor eating habits or destructive patterns of behavior towards food marked by spiritual decay or death?

_____

_____

_____

When I first began to apply the principle of seed sowing to my struggle with food, it seemed a bit silly. After all, it's just food, and wasn't Paul talking about bigger things like bringing people into the kingdom? He was talking about big things, but he was also talking about the multitude of small seeds we plant daily that determine the way we live.

The first seed I planted towards freedom started with preschool. My girls, Brooke and Ally, were two and three years old, and daily I took them to a YMCA preschool down the street. After dropping them off, my habit was to eat continuously until it was time to pick them up. I'd stop by a drive-thru to get a large Diet Coke and wash down handfuls of goldfish, dry cereal, and healthy cookies and crackers. By the time I picked them up, I was stuffed and miserable. As I prayed about the seed I would sow to God in my eating, I decided to sow the time my girls were in preschool. So, after eating a healthy breakfast with them in the morning, I sowed seed from the time I dropped them off to the time I picked them up. From 9:00 to 11:45, rather than grabbing food, I filled myself with praise music, scriptures, and prayer for others. My seed was sown for two hours and forty-five minutes...with no food.

At first it seemed odd. My habits were strong, and I realized mindless eating had consumed my mornings. But after a few days of successful sowing, the seed began to flourish. I looked forward to being intentional rather than mindless, I felt closer to God, and I was excited to sow more seeds throughout the day and evening. It was a start.

As the first week of preschool sowing ended, I added the time I cooked dinner. Normally I'd shove food in my mouth as I prepared a meal and then sit down too full to enjoy it. My next seed was meal prep. During that time, I sowed to the Spirit and offered the hour I prepared food (or less...I'm not a great cook). As I nurtured that seed, I said phrases we've discussed in the previous chapters, like "I don't do that anymore!" as well as affirming scriptures like "I know the truth and the truth is setting me free!"

Let's pause for a moment. Pray right now that the Holy Spirit will show you a seed you can offer to Him for life. Don't skip this. It's the most powerful thing you'll do today. Write the seed offerings that come to mind below.

_____

_____

_____

_____

Now, let's go after the concept of seed sowing from all angles. It isn't just about not doing something. It's about sowing seeds (thoughts, reactions, words, attitudes) that will bring life. There are three areas that seed sowing will dramatically impact:

1. Sowing in rough times of temptation
2. Sowing against the bullies in your mind
3. Sowing to expose secrets

In addition to sowing to stop behaviors we've mindlessly participated in, we sow to win against temptation, to overcome bullies, and to smash secrets we've clung to and protected. Let's look at sowing in rough times of temptation.

Turn to 1 Corinthians 10:13. What does God himself do when you are tempted?

_____

_____

_____

This scripture flips a lot of what we know about temptation on its side. Most of us hunker down in a white-knuckled stance and battle with a gallon of ice cream. This doesn't work! The Greek word for temptation can also mean "test." In the moments our taste buds are saying one thing and our spirit another, we need to view it as a test—a test for which God has given us a cheat sheet to win. Scripture says that all the things that seem tempting to us are common (we tend to think there's something gravely wrong with us and we're the only losers fighting this battle.) It also says God provides a way out. Sowing seed in temptation is listening and acting upon God's exit strategy.

To this day, when I go to a Mexican restaurant, I sow to the Spirit. I love guacamole. I am free to enjoy it, but I have a plan as to how much I will enjoy. Typically, I dip fresh veggies into it rather than chips, but I'm free to have a few chips with it, just not a basket and a half before my meal. There are certain temptation traps we continually fall into. These are the places we're invited to sow to the Spirit for life.
What are some of your temptation traps and how can you offer seed to the Spirit there?

» Time of day I'm most tempted to overeat:

» Type of foods I'm tempted to eat gluttonously:

» Exit strategy God invites me to use:

» Seed I can sow in the midst of this temptation:

Notice that Paul didn't say we'd be free from all temptation. He said God provides an escape, so we can endure it. In other words, God gets us out of there

or teaches us to handle things in the midst of alluring choices—so we are left stronger, better students who have studied this temptation test and know how to pass with flying colors. The more you practice and study sowing seeds in times of temptation, the more you pass the tests.

Friends, remember, this isn't a diet...it's sowing seeds for life. You can't fail or fall off the band wagon. That's old thinking that drives us to despair. When we offer seeds to God, even the smallest seed grows. This is God's promise: **Seeds bear fruit and change the world.** Your world.

Turn to John 15:7-8. What does Jesus promise for those who abide in Him?

_____

_____

What does Jesus say glorifies His Father (vs. 8)?

_____

_____

_____

After we offer seeds for sowing, we need to gently tend to them. As we're intentional to sow seeds, our lives will bear MUCH fruit. Not some...not a little...but much. And boy, how our Father will be glorified.

Tomorrow we'll talk about sowing towards bullies and secrets, but let's end today in 2 Peter 1:2-8. What have we escaped (vs.4) and what is our reward?

_____

_____

_____

Jesus, today I give You seed. It may be small but use it to produce a field of righteousness in my life. Amen.

—— DAY 3: BULLY BASHING AND SECRETS EXPOSED

Jesus, Your peace overcomes the bullies in my mind and the secrets I try to keep. I anxiously wait for Your love. Amen.

My elementary school eventually became my haven, but in first and second grade I was overcome by fear. "Sandy Tipton" was a bully of the worst kind. She was in sixth grade and loved to torture the younger lambs whenever she got the chance. Sadly, I lived on the same block as Sandy, and our bus stop became the scariest place around.

One day, as we were exiting the bus, I must have gotten in her way. The little first graders typically waited until the older kids got off the bus first, but somehow, I accidently broke the protocol. I'll never forget Sandy's mean face. I think she even had a crusty cold sore on her lip! She smashed the books I was holding and they splayed all over the ground. Then she reached out to smack me but when her arm was mid-air, she turned and ran up the hill behind us without delivering the blow. I was so terrified of Sandy I avoided her at all cost—but her bully techniques had everyone in knots.

As I grew older, I became a champion for the underdog or belittled. I now go out of my way to defend them and even in Uganda fight for those who are bullied by corruption. Thank you, Sandy! If I'm honest though, I still fight a bully in my mind (Satan and his minions.) A bully that tries to warp my thinking or push me down—stealing what is truly mine or making me think I don't deserve it. The most powerful way to deal with this bully is by sowing seeds to counteract the bully's antics. Bullies only respond to strength, and sowing seeds in this area will make us strong.

Please turn to Deuteronomy 30:14-16. Write verse 14 below.

_____

_____

_____

_____

I love this verse because it states what's true when a bully threatens to strike. "The word is very near you; it is in your mouth and in your heart so you may obey it." Moses continues by reminding us the Lord is blessing us in the land we are entering so we can possess it...not so we can sit by and let a bully dominate us! To possess new land there's usually a battle for the title. Whoever owns the title owns the land. As you sow seeds against mind bullies, you are literally taking new land—and the title of ownership is completely yours in Jesus Christ.

Now let's look at Deuteronomy 30:19-20. What are the two "seed" choices set before us (vs. 19)? What happens when we sow seeds to life?

_____

_____

_____

We know God gives us the choice to sow towards life in our thoughts. For those of us who've been around a while, we're sure scripture is the punch that knocks the voice out of a bully. The problem is sometimes we forget how to throw the punch. Perhaps life has been rough, or we've experienced a season of disappointment. In these times it's easy to get cynical—or doubt the power we have to sow seed. This is why it's important to remember how a bully thinks:

1. A bully sees you as weak.
2. A bully assumes a posture of dominance.
3. A bully is afraid to lose power, so they hurt those they feel they can control.

Sowing seeds to the Spirit crushes each of these postures because truth is a weapon that sets the captive free. Read the following and then note how the scriptures fight the mind bullies we face.

Smirks or blows of a bully:

- I can't overcome this challenge.
- I'm not smart enough, pretty enough, talented enough.
- This is the best it can be. I have to accept it.
- My best days have passed.
- I'm invisible and, unlovable, and I don't have purpose.
- God's ways are too hard to make sense of. I've tried to trust but see nothing change.

Seeds to sow against the blows: (Note how these apply to your personal bully attacks, and add more of your own.)

- 2 Corinthians 10:4: _____
- Deuteronomy 20:1-4: _____
- Isaiah 40:29: _____
- Psalm 22:19: _____

Now let's talk about secrets. Once I was teaching at a First Place for Health gathering and after teaching about freedom from "secret eating," a woman approached and said she had no problems in this area. As a matter of fact, she thought it was a bit strange. I smiled politely, and as she turned to walk away she stopped abruptly and said, "I just thought of something maybe I should share. Last week as I was driving home from the grocery store I reached for the package of cookies I'd bought. They were the chocolate, vanilla, and strawberry wafers I love. I thought I'd only eat one or two of the chocolate—but by the time I got home I'd eaten the whole package, and I hid the wrappers, so my husband wouldn't see or ask. Do you think that's secret eating?"

The truth is, many of us are unaware we spend a lot of time planning how to eat without anyone seeing us or noticing. I was the queen of secret eating. People would say, "You're the healthiest eater I know!" as I'd nibble on a green salad with no dressing. Then, at home in the back pantry I'd shovel handfuls of cereal, bread, or leftover mac and cheese into my mouth while no one was looking. The charade was, "If no one sees, it doesn't count." Or, "I don't want anyone to see my out-of-control choices, so I'll eat like this only in secret." This is why drive-thrus are an overeater's best friend. You can pull up to a metal box, order a lot of food, eat in the peace of your car—and no one sees. The lure of a secret tryst lasts only for a moment, and then the realization that something's wrong settles in.

When I began to sow healthy seeds to secret eating, I was terrified but full of resolve. The first seed I sowed was in the evenings. Typically, Bobby would have a small bowl of ice cream as we relaxed after getting the kids to bed. I'd never eat ice cream with him because I was too healthy of an eater (so he thought). Yet, I'd sneak food secretly while he peacefully ate his treat. The night I began sowing to secrets I dished him out a few scoops of ice cream, and instead of sneaking around, I dished myself a scoop too. Then I sat down on the couch with him like a normal person and ate the ice cream without secrets or compulsion. Because I was sowing to the Spirit, I didn't go back for more bites secretly, and I didn't feel the need to eat ice cream all day the next day. The word from Philippians 4:13 rang through my head, "I can do all this through him who gives me strength." As I began to sow seeds to secret eating, the desire to hide in the shadows with food lost its appeal. Never again did I eat secretly in shame. The power of secrets is the isolation in which they're kept. Once a secret is exposed, it loses its power.

Do you see any patterns of secrecy in your eating? Would you be ashamed if your family, a friend, or Jesus himself saw you eating in certain settings?

_____

_____

_____

Proverbs 9:17-18 (NIV) says, "'Stolen water is sweet; food eaten in secret is delicious!' But little do they know that the dead are there, that her guests are deep in the realm of dead." These verses are talking about the lure of a loose woman trying to capture an innocent man, but the reference to food is powerful. Why does eating secretly seem sweet and delicious?

_____

_____

_____

What kind of good seed can you sow to secret eating today? Be specific as you write down and describe the seed you'll sow.

_____

_____

_____

Jesus, You are the light of the world. Where You go, light follows. I want Your light in the secrets of my behaviors and in the bully-driven thoughts that flood my mind. Amen.

—— DAY 4: GIVING YOUR BEST

Lord, You gave Your best for me on the cross. I give my best toYyou as I sow seeds towards new life. Amen.

When I was young, we used to give things up around the season of Lent. The whole idea was to present a sacrifice in remembrance of the sacrifice Jesus made for humanity on the cross. Typically, we gave up some kind of food—which seemed really hard as a child. One year I figured I'd out-smart the system. I gave up popcorn, which in theory sounds nice, but truthfully, I rarely had the opportunity to eat popcorn except for at the movies, which I almost never attended. We didn't have a popcorn maker, so the sacrifice was pretty much a sham. It wasn't until Easter that I realized I'd only been fooling myself. As I reflected on the joy I could have had if I'd offered something meaningful, I wished I could have gone back and done a "do-over." That's the beauty of Jesus: he constantly gives second chances if we're committed to giving our best.

When it comes to sowing seeds with food and setting ourselves up for success in what we offer, Paul teaches powerfully on the way we sow.

Turn to 2 Corinthians 9:6-7. How did Paul describe the way we sow?

_____

_____

Paul used two words to describe how we shouldn't sow—reluctantly or under compulsion. Many of my pre-freedom attempts to manage my behavior with food were rife with compulsion. I either ate out-of-control or dieted with obsessive control. Compulsion leads to obsession, and reluctance leads to bitter resolve. Neither points towards freedom, let alone a cheerful disposition.

In your past relationship with food, can you note times of reluctance or compulsion as you've tried to deal with this problem? Explain.

_____
_____
_____

Let's continue in these verses. Read 2 Corinthians 9:10-11. Who gives you the seed you'll sow and what happens to that seed?

_____
_____
_____

It's God who gives us seed to sow. Not only does He give us the seed as we sow generously, He increases the amount of seeds we get to sow back to Him and brings a great reward in the sowing. It reminds me of giving our small children money to buy Christmas presents. On Christmas we unwrap something they've lovingly given, but ultimately, we were the ones who provided the means for the gift. Every seed we sow already belongs to God. Our obedience and heart for free-dom are rightfully His, but He provides opportunities for us to give it back to Him as a gift. That's why it's so important to decide to sow abundantly not sparingly. We want to bless God and reap generously in return.

In what ways can you sow generously this week? Think of timeframes, secrets, or thoughts you want to change. Don't be skimpy on what you offer. Remember,

God loves a cheerful giver, and He blesses and returns everything we sow in a rich harvest.

_____
_____
_____

Please turn to Mark 4:26-29. How did Mark describe the process of a seed's growth?

_____

_____

_____

This parable is recorded only by Mark. It's not seen in the other gospels, which is fitting, because Mark loved to explain the words of Jesus in a clear and forthright way. In these verses Jesus re-vealed that spiritual growth is an on-going, continual process that gradually ends in maturity. Once our seed has ripened and grown, it produces a harvest of maturity.

Now let's finish with Jesus's words in Mark 4:30-32. These are my favorite words regarding seeds in the entire Bible. What inspires you in these verses?

_____

_____

_____

_____

I have a small bottle of mustard seeds on the shelf in my office. The seeds are only the size of a pin-top, but Jesus says size doesn't matter. In the end, these small seeds produce one of the largest trees known. What a perfect reminder that even if our seeds are small, they are powerful.   Small seeds might look like times of the day you offer to God for praise rather than food intake. It might look like sowing a scripture out loud, rather than repeating a lie the bully (Satan) repeatedly screams in your head. Or, it might look like training your taste buds to truly enjoy food that's healthy, one broccoli stem at a time. Whatever the seed, it's precious to God, and He multiplies it to your harvest.

Father, You are the seed giver and the seed tender. In Your abundant care, I reap a harvest of blessing as I continue to offer You my seed. I long to give You more. Amen.

—— DAY 5: IT'S MORE THAN JUST A SEED

Lord, I know that as I give more of myself to You, You make me more like You. There's nothing I desire more in life than this. Amen.

This week we've studied the principle of sowing seeds and seen how it impacts our lives and choices. Today, I want to share a new outlook on seeds that outshines anything else we know.

Seed sowing is an act of worship.

Too often we see worship as the songs we sing in church or the playlist we listen to on our drive to work. Worship is so much more than songs—it's the acknowledgment that God is our breath, our love, and our purpose. It's an act of humility and awe that brings us into communion with Father, Son and Holy Spirit. True worship quietly gives itself over to holiness because the more we worship, the holier we become.

When we plant seeds in our lives as an offering to God, it's a sacred act of worship. We worship as we believe for change. We worship as we bow in obedience to the death of a voracious appetite that food was never meant to satisfy.

Perhaps it's time we shift our understanding. Every seed we sow is an act of worship.

Please turn to Luke 8:4-8. Although you may be familiar with this theme, read the parable with a new lens. What four types of sowing were described by Jesus? Where were the seeds sown and what happened to the seed?

Verse 5:

Verse 6:

Verse 7:

Verse 8:

Now let's try to put these seed sowing categories to use in our own behavior and choices. Can you recall periods of trying new diets, programs, or food plans, only to see your efforts trampled or wither away? How did it make you feel about yourself?

_____

_____

_____

Have you ever lost weight successfully, only to regain or return to habits you tried to overcome? Explain how you felt as old habits you thought you were rid of choked out the new habits you tried so hard to establish.

_____

_____

_____

Now read Jesus's words in Luke 8:11-15. What's the seed?

_____

_____

So, the word of God is planted in the soil of our lives and the devil (the bully) is at work to steal and trample it so it won't bear fruit. In rocky soil our seed has no root, and when we're tempted, we immediately fail.

When the seed is planted in soil with thorns, the worry and pleasures of life ("I really want to eat lots of this...what's the big deal?") choke out the power of the seed to grow. But seeds planted in good soil represent those who have listened with an honest and pure heart. They hold the seed tightly and offer it in worship. They bear fruit when they don't give up.

No one in their right mind would say "I want to fail! I want to be weak and languish in immaturity!" Yet, so many of us continue to plant seeds this way. True worship offers something different.

Let's look at this from another perspective. Turn to Genesis 4:1-5. What words would you use to describe Abel and Cain?

_____

_____

_____

_____

It's no accident that Abel was both the first recorded shepherd and the first martyr for worshipping God in truth. It's also interesting that this drama ultimately revolved around food and the way it was offered.

Both men were given a way (seed) to offer back to the Lord. One man gave of his best while the other gave a sloppy offering. Listen to the simplicity of these words: "Abel was a shepherd while Cain was a farmer. At harvest time Cain brought the Lord a gift of his farm produce, and Abel brought the fatty cuts of meat from his best lambs and presented them to the Lord."[2]

The Bible doesn't say Cain gave no offering. It just highlights that his brother Abel gave the best animals he raised, while Cain brought the average or least amount he had to, so he could say he offered something to the Lord. How many times do we offer God a token rather than our best when we sow seeds for change? Considering it's an act of worship—let's hope we never do it again.

Read verses 6-7. How did God continue to pursue Cain? What did he say to him about sin?

It's so like God to try in every way he can to help us see things from the right perspective. He practically shakes Cain and says "Sin is ready to take you down. Jealousy and envy are blinding you, but you can overcome this and be happy! You can win this battle!"

Ultimately, Cain was dealing with more that just offering sloppy seconds. Rather than truly interacting with God as he sowed seeds of worship, he had his eyes on the gifts of his brother, making him envy the favor God had for his sibling. Even seed sowing can be tainted if we take our eyes off the one who receives the seed we sow.

Have you ever felt jealous of someone who seems to have no trouble with food? Envious of someone who has a great body or has had success with weight loss as you continue to struggle?

Even a seed sown in honesty is a seed that can flourish. God told Cain he'd be bright with joy if he did what he should to bring the right offering. It was a heart matter not a fruit matter. Is there a heart seed you need to give to the Lord today as an act of worship? Perhaps there's someone you're jealous of who seems to glide through life, while you struggle with difficult obstacles (health, relationships, weight, finances).

Or perhaps you've been holding back on giving the Lord your best because you don't want to fail, or truthfully, don't want to give up what you like to consume and how you like to consume it. Please explain below.

Today we leave behind old seed and offer new seed as an act of worship. After you read this description below, please shut your eyes for a moment and pray.

Lord, we take in our hands a seed offering. This offering looks like poor choices with food, doubting attitudes, cynical outlooks, and a foreboding sense that we'll never change. Right now, we are throwing these seeds behind us, for they are incapable of new growth. We take up new seed and plant it in the soil of a broken heart. The soil of our hearts has been tilled and turned over, ready for good seed. As we nurture the seed and help it grow, we offer this to You as an act of worship. It's not a matter of willpower or might, but of surrender to the power of the seed and trust in the One who makes it grow. Amen.

—— DAY 6: REFLECTION AND APPLICATION
Lord Jesus, You are the Vine, and we are merely Your branches. You give life as we surrender to Your ways of growth. Amen.

Recently I spoke to a group of women about the power of seeds. I was teaching on the sunflower and how they grow from small seeds to plants that tower over six feet tall. The sunflower remarkably follows the scientific pattern of phototropism—which means throughout the day the face of the flower stretches towards the sun. The plant literally shifts positions as it follows the light and warmth of what causes it to grow. What a beautiful picture of how we can live our lives, moving throughout the day to face our Son.

The seeds of the sunflower grow in the center of the flower. They fall off and quickly spread as birds and the wind whisk them away to new surroundings, causing new sunflowers to spring up where the seeds have been taken.

After I delivered this message, I handed hundreds of women their own little packet of sunflower seeds. They could plant them or simply keep them as a reminder to follow the Son and to be scattered as the seed that falls from the abundance of the flower brings nutrition and new beauty wherever it grows.

This weekend buy a packet of seeds from the grocery store, or simply put a small container of sunflower seeds on your counter for a few weeks. Use these as a reminder of the power of sowing seeds.

Lord, I know You bring great reward from seed offered in truth and hope. I offer You the seed of expectation. I renounce all negativity and the attitudes that keep me stuck or bored. Amen.

—— DAY 7: REFLECTION AND APPLICATION

Lord, as I pray to You, show me the fields to be sown and the seeds I can offer to You as worship. Amen.

This week we talked about the difference between sowing generously (without reluctance or compulsion) and sowing sparingly (not sure we'll succeed so we hold back). Talk to your prayer partner about whatever holds you back from sowing with a new and excited heart. Remember, seed sowing is not dieting. Dieting sets us up for failure as it implies a list of rules and regulations that must be followed. Seed sowing is active and alive. It's lifegiving and full of hope. Seed sowing is an act of worship.

Discuss this one question with your prayer partner and circle back to it each day this week:

How can I sow seeds of worship in my life?

Note: Your seeds can be about anything you want to offer to the Lord. They do not have to exclusively center around food but can be anything you'd like to bring new life and change to (fear, worry, bitterness, anxiety, criticism, anger, loneliness, laziness, loosening control over things we aren't meant to hold on to). Use your prayer partner as a friend and fellow sower who understands the process you're going through.

Jesus, my seeds fall on a true soil of worship. I willingly plant for You. Amen.

Notes

1. Gari Meacham, Be Free (Galveston, Tex.: First Place for Health, 2017), 95.
2. TLB Life Application Bible (Carol Stream, Ill.,: Tyndale House Publishers, 2012), 13.

WEEK SIX: TIME FOR HARVEST

SCRIPTURE MEMORY VERSE

He told them, "The harvest is plentiful, but the workers are few. Ask the Lord of the harvest, therefore, to send out workers into his harvest field."
Luke 10: 2

The beautiful man my daughter Brooke married is a winemaker in Sonoma Valley. He's in charge of making one of the finest wines in the country—which means his life ebbs and flows with the rhythm of the grapes. Harvest occurs during the months of September through November, and for a few long months the physical and mental strain of turning grapes into wine rivals running five consecutive marathons. (At least that's how he describes it!)

We like to think of harvest as a romantic time. A time of lush baskets filled with bountiful fruit. But the truth is...harvest is hard. It's the culmination of months and sometimes years—of hard, intentional work. After sowing seeds and nurturing their growth, we arrive at harvest, anxious to glean the reward of our efforts. The problem is reaping rewards can be illusive. When it comes to living *Beyond Free*—what does harvest look like? Losing twenty pounds? Keeping weight off for more than a year? Forgoing the insanity of yo-yo dieting and making peace with our compulsive ways?

Jesus said something profound when He talked about the harvest. He said there's a plentiful harvest waiting but those who can bring it in are few. We know that He was discussing the harvest of souls and salvation, but I believe He was also laying a foundation for deeper meaning. Prior to these verses Jesus was teaching a wave of lessons on what it means to be a disciple. He talked about not getting caught in prejudice squabbles (Luke 9:54) and following him no matter the cost (vs. 62.) Then, while preparing to send them out into cities He would soon visit, He spoke of the ripe harvest. He explained that lives are ready, but there aren't enough people mature enough or willing to do the hard work of harvest (Luke 10:2). Thus, potential and the chance for wonderful growth are left on the vine.

We've learned how to sow seeds to the Spirit for life and how to sow generously, not sparingly. In the pages ahead, we'll learn that harvest comes from the success of obedience. Together, we're both mature enough and willing to work for a rich reward.

—— DAY 1: IT PAYS TO OBEY

Jesus, I tend to view obedience as a chore, when truthfully, it's a gift. Help me to willingly give this gift to You today. Amen.

The concept of obedience has gotten a bad rap. We tend to think of it as a nuisance rather than an invitation to something great—another opportunity to fail God and not hold up our end of the bargain. But here's the rub: we never get to harvest if we don't first lean into what it means to obey. To obey God isn't to be chained to unrealistic standards and expectations. On the contrary. To obey God is to hear God and act accordingly. Holman's Illustrated Bible Dictionary says, "Obedience means to hear, trust, submit, and surrender to God and his word." We understand hearing from God and his Word; it's the trust, submission and surrender that give us trouble.

Can we be honest? We need to quit thinking obedience is optional and start viewing it as essential. When it comes to food and our appetites, it's a win-win when we commit to His ways.

So, let's look at a few reasons it's essential to obey.

Jesus says to.
Read John 14:15. How does Jesus make this plain?

_____

_____

_____

Most of us would readily admit we love Jesus. Yet, He tells us to follow His command to love one another as we love ourselves (Mark 12:31) I know many men and women who are brutal to themselves yet loving to others. The other day I was mentally badgering myself for who knows what when I quietly heard the peaceful voice of the Spirit say, "You're a good woman, Gari." I almost had to pull over to the side of the road and weep. It'd been a long while since I felt that way. What a joy it was to be reminded in such a gentle way. Friends, if you've been telling yourself what a failure you are with food or obedience as a whole, maybe it's time for you to obey Jesus and show yourself some love.

Obedience is worship.
Read Romans 12:1. What did Paul say is pleasing to God?

_____

_____

When was the last time you viewed obedience as a living sacrifice, not something routine or dead? Your obedience is holy and pleasing to God. If you're in an obedience rut, break out and roam the vast fields of freedom. You get to make good choices instead of have to.

Now turn to Romans 6:11-13. What does verse 13 say we must stop doing?

_____

_____

_____

One translation says, "...and do not go on presenting the members of your body to sin as instruments of unrighteousness; but present yourselves to God as alive from the dead, and your members as instruments of righteousness to God" (NASB, emphasis added). Here is a play on words: instead of presenting parts of our bodies to sin, we can offer them as a present to God for righteousness.
What parts of your body are you presenting to sin rather than righteousness? (Think: mouth, eyes, hands, feet, stomach.)

_____

_____

How can you shift this behavior to worship as you obey?

_____

_____

God rewards obedience.
Turn to James 1:22-25. What happens when we listen to God's Word but don't do what it says to do?

_____

_____

_____

James reminds us that if we look intently towards the freedom God gives and live it out, we'll be blessed in what we do. There's great reward for those who obey.

I mentioned in our week's introduction that harvest is the success of obedience. It's the sum of all the intentional choices we make and seeds we sow. Many of us are in a continual season of planting (sticking to things for a while but never following through, mustering up resolve only to fall away after an initial burst of hope to change). It's good to plant and sow seeds, but we must *bring things to a harvest* if we're ever to experience the reward.

What things have you started (planted and sown) in the past six months that have never come to a harvest? Reflect on all areas of your life, not just those having to do with food. This could be any activity you've started and stopped or dreams you began to pursue but quit because they got hard.

Now let's commit to a harvest. Where do you long to see reward? Are there things you've begun but never finished? Dreams you once had that seem impossible? Commit these things to the Lord of the Harvest. Ask Him to strengthen you as you obey with new vigor. Harvest begins with seeds that have ripened. It's your season to bring things from seedling to fruition. Write a prayer of commitment towards harvest below.

My Harvest Commitment:

Jesus, You are the Lord of the harvest. I long for my life to be white with blossoms. Amen.

—— DAY 2: SONGS OF HARVEST
Father, I hear the song of my harvest. Let me sing with expectant joy. Amen.

Please turn to Psalm 126:1-6. Write verse 6 below.

This psalm is part of the Psalms of Ascent sung by the Jews as they walked toward the temple in worship. Like us, they experienced the disappointment and frustration of life, but they set their minds and voices to a harvest. The picture of weeping as we sow seeds is so tender. It's a reminder that everything we set our minds to do in obedience, no matter how small or seemingly insignificant, matters to God. As a matter of fact, God guarantees we will return from sowing with songs of joy, carrying the outcome of what we've sown.

Now let's focus on verse one of this psalm. The NIV translation says, "When the Lord restored the fortunes of Zion, we were like those who dreamed." For some of us, it's been a long time since we dreamed. It may seem as though dreams are for younger men and women and that our fate is sealed. This couldn't be farther from the truth. The Lord restores what's been taken from us. For some, this means a restoration of your identity, health, confidence, stamina, and ability to function in a sharp and productive way. For others it means a restoration of dignity if you've been abused, clarity if you've been betrayed, and hope if you've been disappointed.

Is there something you need restored today—enabling you to dream again?

_____

_____

_____

What does God say our response will be in Psalm 126:2?

_____

_____

_____

Sowing seeds, especially when it feels hard, can be challenging. Oswald Chambers explains this beautifully:

> "'They that sow in tears...'—it looks as though the seed were drowned. You can see the seed when it's in the basket, but when it falls into the ground, it disappears. The seed is the word of God, and no word of God is ever fruitless. If I know that the sowing is going to bring forth fruit, I am blessed in the drudgery. Drudgery is never blessed, but drudgery can be enlightened."

Perhaps if we remember the enlightenment of drudgery, we'll know that God is looking after every menial task and difficult choice with the prize of understanding and growth.

Now please turn to Isaiah 21: 10. What does the prophet call God's people and where does he say they are?

_____

_____

_____

Isaiah says God's people are crushed on the threshing floor. He has spoken of the fall of Babylon with their false idols, but describes God's people as threshed and winnowed in the wake.

In the farming process of ancient Israel, the threshing and winnowing happened in two steps. "The heads of wheat were first trampled to break open the seeds and expose the valued grain inside. The seeds were then thrown into the air and the worthless chaff blew away while the grain fell back to the ground."[1] Too often, we stop at the process of threshing. Our lives and habits are exposed, and God is winnowing away what is worthless. If we let the threshing takes its course, we'll reap a harvest.

Some of us have never gotten off the threshing floor. We quit after things are exposed and roll around in the worthless chaff, while some of us have been living free of the bad chaff but want more of the good grain. Instead, we should strive for more maturity, more growth, more harvest,

In the book of Ruth, we see a beautiful picture of threshing, gleaning and harvest. Please turn to Ruth 2:1-23. How did God use the process of reaping and gleaning to take Ruth to a new place of joy in her life?

_____

_____

_____

It's important to remember that gleaning the leftover wheat and barley in the fields was hard, humiliating work. Ruth's husband was gone, and she and her mother-in-law were considered the poorest of the poor in society as widows. Gleaning on the fields was a type of welfare system she was not too proud to try. Through her willingness to glean and allow the grain she gathered to be threshed, her entire future changed as her relative Boaz recognized her inner beauty and became a kinsman redeemer—to marry and protect her. From her obedience in the fields, she became a mother in the lineage of Jesus.

Father, we don't always see the benefit of life's threshing, but You always bring a harvest. Like Ruth, help us to patiently and willingly do the work. Amen.

—— DAY 3: PROTECTING THE HARVEST

Lord, we ask You to guard what we work so hard to achieve. Protect our harvest with Your hedge and holy fire. Amen.

In biblical days a hedge protected grape vineyards. A hedge was either a tight-branched bush or a special kind of fence built to serve as a barrier. This barrier kept bugs, rodents, birds, and thieves from entering or stealing from the vineyard. In spiritual terms, a hedge is the promise of God's protection for those who love and walk with Him. A hedge is something we can pray for and continue to build as we seek protection for the things we've worked so hard to nurture and grow.

One of the most popular mentions of a hedge is in the book of Job. Please turn to Job 1:10-12. How did Satan describe the relationship Job has with God? What was God's response?

Most translations use word hedge to describe the protective hand of God. Basically, Satan said, "Sure, anyone would love you, God, if they had the blessing and protection you've given Job." In this moment, God was so sure of Job's character and future that he allowed the hedge to be removed temporarily, so that Satan has access to his life's vineyard. One pastor described this perplexing scene so well: "God's protective hand is so powerful over our lives. I wonder what would happen if it was removed completely?"

Job understood the concept of spiritual protection. As a matter of fact, it's what set him apart.

Read Job 1:4-5. What did Job do regularly regarding his children?

Job made a regular practice of getting up early and sacrificing on behalf of his children. He prayed a covering over them in case there were any sins they'd committed unknowingly. According to Bible history, Job arose as early as 4:30 to intercede this protection around his children. God honored his conviction and earnestness— and even in his period of greatest testing and loss, God protected Job's faith from bitterness.

When it comes to protecting what we've worked hard for (new habits, new behaviors, healthy life change) or the things we love, it's wise, like Job, to ask for a hedge of protection to be placed around us.

To understand the concept of hedges further, let's study several scriptures that show more about their power and purpose.

The Hedge of Peace
Read Philippians 4:8-9. What type of thinking did Paul say will bring God's protective peace to us?

_____

_____

_____

_____

The Hedge of Understanding
Read Psalm 119:33-37. How did the psalmist ask for greater understanding? What kind of things does understanding protect us from?

_____

_____

_____

The Hedge of Angelic Protection
Turn to Psalm 34:4-7. How do God's angels serve as protection for you?

_____

_____

_____

Read Psalm 91:11-12. What does God command his angels to do on your behalf?

_____

_____

The Hedge of Hope

Read Romans 15: 13. What happens as we are hedged in by hope?

Our lives are protected by hedges put in place by God's loving care and by our tenacious belief in His power to oversee our circumstances and growth.

What are you most afraid of losing? Why do you think that fear is so prevalent?

Praying for God's protection takes away fear of the unknown and places trust in the love God has for us—his children. So often, we spend more time worrying about things that might happen than praying for the protection and authority of God to overcome it. It's important to remember that when bad things happen, it's not God's punishment or lack of power. He is always at work, crafting a mosaic that may not make sense on earth but does in eternity. Don't forget: the enemy's goal is pain and confusion while God's is wisdom and love.

Remember the vineyard and the harvest? Farmers would guard their treasure at all cost. There were several layers of protection guarding the crops until harvest was complete, but what I love the most is the fire built in the vineyard just before harvest. The fire was to purge the area of flying insects or birds that would get in the way when the fruit was picked. Author Ron Phillips describes it like this:

"We arrive at harvest time when the grapes are ripe, following the long season during which we have waited, and waited, and waited. The Father has watched over us, but now the fruit is ripe, and the fragrance is wafting. It's when we are at the point of reaping the greatest blessings in our lives that every demon of hell, every insect and fowl bird wants to lodge in the branches! But God says, 'I'm sending Holy Spirit fire.' And when that fire begins to burn, the smoke of His glory rises, and nothing can come and get our harvest."

Satan has ruined many harvests, but what we've spent time sowing is worth protecting. He cannot penetrate the powerful hedge of God. Pray for the things you've spiritually worked hard for and for the people you love. Your harvest is here.

Dear Father,
I pray Your protective hedge over my life right now. I ask You to set a bordering hedge around my spouse, my children, my home, my health, my mind, my finances—and everything I love. I pray this not out of fear, but from a heart of trust. I am Your child, and You are a good Father who delights in my love. Life on earth is challenging, but remind me that earth is not my home—heaven is. As I trust in You, I reap a bountiful harvest. Set Your holy fire ablaze in my vineyard, purging my life of anything that might try to steal the fullness of my fruit. With love and praise, amen.

—— DAY 4: THE NEXT RIGHT THING

Jesus, I always want to listen and obey, but the truth is...I don't. Help me to honestly face my actions and choose the next right thing without wallowing in defeat. Amen.

We've been studying sowing seeds and reaping a harvest, which sounds beautiful and lyrical, but suddenly, I'm reminded of the vast world of gray—the decisions and choices that aren't black and white, but rather, a deep shade of in-between. Should I eat this? Did I eat too much? How do I get back on track after a fatty dinner, a milkshake, and a half-pound of Oreos? Double stuffed. These are the questions that must be answered when it comes to obedience as we vacillate in the gray land.

One of my good friends at First Place for Health, Becky Turner, says, "Do the next right thing." Wow...that's wise. There's so much teaching and hype around succeeding—but what happens when you don't? What do you do when you failed to make good choices...perhaps for weeks, months, or years? How do you set things straight? The answer is clear—do the next right thing.

The moments *after you've failed* are the most powerful opportunities to grow. In these moments we have two options. We can either throw our hands up and say, "What's the use?" Or, we can instantly speak to God and sow a good seed by vowing to leave the poor choice behind and make a good choice right then and there. Sowing seed in moments of defeat brings God into these moments rather than shutting him out. And where God is, there is peace.

Please turn to James 1:12-17. What happens when we make poor choices (vs. 14-15)?

_____

_____

Where does every good thing come from (vs. 17)?

_____

_____

I used to have a friend who struggled with bulimia. It was so extreme she found herself throwing up several times a day. When she heard me talk about sowing seeds and obedience, she confessed she thought she was too far gone for any of this to work. So, we came up with a plan. Every time she walked into the bathroom, instead of shutting God out, she invited him in. Even if she found herself slumped over the toilet, she continued to speak to God instead of hiding spiritually. In the moments after she succumbed to her destructive choice, she offered her heart and the next minutes to God for praise and new resolve. She confessed she was partnering with death and invited the Father of Light to fill the room with the good gifts He longed to give her.

Over the course of the next two weeks, several trips to the bathroom diminished to one, and soon, what used to be a time of destruction became a seed of praise. She no longer made ANY trips to throw up—and began to share her hope with other young girls living in defeat. She chose to do the next right thing.

Let's study this a bit further. Please turn to these scriptures and answer the questions below.

Ephesians 4:22-24: What should we do with our old self? What's glaringly different about the old self and the new?

_____

_____

_____

Deuteronomy 8:3: Why does overeating, binging, over-controlling or obsessing about food leave us empty? What are we really meant to be sustained by?

_____

_____

_____

Psalm 73:25-26: What can we count on when our flesh and heart fail?

Sowing good seed in our poor choices is every bit as important as sowing in the good times. The longer we let a poor choice fester, the more it's given the chance to shove us down.

I knew I was moving towards freedom when times of defeat and toe-to-toe battles with temptation started to diminish in frequency. Here's a sampling of how I sowed to the Spirit rather than spinning into a dark cycle of defeat.

After eating 12 cookies rather than the two I'd set aside, I offered this seed to the Lord:

"Father, I planned on making a better choice in this moment. I even set aside what I planned to eat as I baked rather than leaving it to chance...but instead, I scarfed food down simply because it tasted good in those split seconds. From this new moment on, I will honor You in my choices and not continue down a binging path. I ask You into this timeframe, to fill me with a new peace in this new moment. I'm walking away from this food and will praise You in the next few steps I take."

I'm not one to bash comfort food because I think food was created to be enjoyed and even to be a comfort at times. Where this gets tricky is when it becomes a habitual pacifier rather than the comfort of God. Here's my seed for those moments:

"Lord, Your Word says that you are my refuge and source of strength, not food. I'm free to enjoy food, but my true hope is in You not something I put in my mouth. I choose to move out of food comfort this minute (leave the kitchen, pantry, wherever I'm eating) and rest in You, even if it feels strange, as Your comfort is real."

Some seeds are action oriented rather than prayer-like. If I find myself reaching for food when I'm not hungry or mindlessly eating without intention, my seed is to physically replace the eating with a different behavior. When I was breaking free, I'd often go walk the block and give myself a certain timeframe when I wouldn't pick up food until the allotted time was over. If it was late afternoon, I might have said, "I'm mindlessly eating right now, so I'm going to get out of this house and go walk the block as I praise." (Or walk the backyard, organize my closet, call a friend.) Even when I've made a poor choice (eating without intention), I would turn my poor choice into something that brings life.

What are some seeds you can pre-plan to offer so you can do the next right thing after you've made a poor choice?

Let's close by reading Psalm 119:129-133. Write the words of verse 133 below and make it your prayer today.

Lord Jesus, I don't want to let any sin have dominion over me. In the moments I feel trapped or frustrated, I sow seed to You and to life. Amen.

—— DAY 5: HARVEST IS HERE

Jesus, You are Lord of the Harvest and Lord of my life. All that I've sown is Yours. Amen.

One of the frustrating things for me as an author is to see people grow, thrive, and change...for a while. For some reason, after we see positive results or a movement of God, we slip back into the dead end behaviors we begged to be free from! In our discussion of seed sowing—it's like planting seeds, nurturing their growth, and finally, when the harvest is ready to be reaped—leaving ripe fruit on the vines.

Friends, we're not leaving any fruit on the vine! You've worked too hard. And even if your harvest is smaller than you'd like, it's still a harvest to celebrate.

Please turn to Zechariah 8:12. Describe what the prophet said will happen to the seed, the vine, and the land.

Now turn to Leviticus 26:3-5. What does verse 5 say will happen if we follow God's commands?

_____

_____

_____

Both Moses and Zechariah speak of an assurance of God's favor as we sow and harvest in the safe way he intends. The NIV translation puts it this way: "Your threshing will continue until grape harvest and grape harvest will continue until planting, and *you will eat all the food you want and live in safety in your land*" (*Leviticus 26:5, emphasis added*).

Is God saying we can eat like an all-you-can-eat buffet and nothing will harm us? No. He's saying that when we do it *His* way (sane choices, following His command to grow in the fruit of self-discipline, offering our bodies as a living and holy sacrifice), then we live in the safety of the land.

Now read Leviticus 26:9-10. What is the result of God's favor in these verses?

_____

_____

_____

I love the fact that as we sow seeds of obedience to God, He increases our harvest! So much so, that each year of obedience the harvest multiplies so quickly we can't even finish the fruit of the last year before the bountiful treasure of the new year overtakes it.

When I began to live *Beyond Free*, it was amazing how much mental capacity I had for kingdom thoughts rather than thoughts revolving around food. As God increases your harvest, you may find yourself in wonderfully unfamiliar territory. But to get there, you need to remove any thoughts keeping you from your harvest.

Has your weight kept you from doing something you'd love to do? (This is a harvest blocker.)

_____

_____

_____

Does your attachment to food outweigh your desire to obey God's plan for health? (This is a harvest blocker.)

Do you find yourself thinking things will never change—that hope is for others but not for you? (This is a harvest blocker.)

Is there something specific you know is blocking your harvest? Describe it below.

If you know there are things blocking your harvest, today is the day we'll remove them.

Please turn back to Zechariah 9:11-12. What does God promise to do (vs. 11)?

What does he promise to restore?

Zechariah is known as the prophet who specifically and supernaturally described the movements of the coming Messiah. In a powerful play on words, the prophet assures that because of the blood of his covenant, the prisoners are free from the waterless pit. Jesus is the living water that lifts us like a wave out of any pit we crawl into. He promises his truth sets us free, and the blood of his covenant seals it.

Then, like a stunning ending to a great plot, the prophet said, "Return to the strong-hold, O prisoners who have the hope; this very day I am declaring that I will restore double to you" (Zechariah 9:12 NASB, emphasis added).

In biblical days the word stronghold meant the protective place of God. The prophet is telling us to return to the protective place of God and he will restore double what we've lost.

Imagine walking double the miles you walk? Double the good night's sleep you enjoy? Double the meaningful conversations and Gospel impact? Double the seeds you sow towards righteousness? Double your peace and confidence? This isn't some name-it-claim-it scheme—it's a promise of restoration from the Lord. If we continue to return to the safety of God's way, he'll double our harvest.

Jesus, I don't want an average life with You; I want an abundant life. Help me to see the difference. Amen.

—— DAY 6: REFLECTION AND APPLICATION

Lord, thank You for new perspective. Sometimes a shift in thinking makes the biggest difference in my life. I love You. Amen.

This week we've looked at the word harvest in a personal way. The whole notion of sowing seeds and reaping the reward of obedience is exciting—but Jesus takes the concept a step further. Ultimately, there's a purpose beyond our own sanctification (a scary sounding word that simply means the process of becoming holy). The purpose is a harvest of souls. In a stunning encounter in the book of John, Jesus invites us to a harvest of remarkable proportion: "Behold, I say to you, lift up your eyes and look on the fields, that they are white for harvest" (John 4:35).

It's daunting when we try to conjure up ways to go get souls. Truthfully, that never works. What seems to be far more effective is using our brokenness to invite others into a safe and welcoming fold. At speaking events when I share my story of food compulsion, struggle, and how it led me to the Savior, Jesus Christ, it's beautiful to see how authenticity is better than scholarly knowledge. When we're open about our struggles rather than hiding them, we gain access into the heart of people strug-gling with the same issues—and we point them to a Savior who has answers to every question and heartfelt sigh. It's then we become a planter and reaper in the harvest of souls.

Reflect today on ways you can use your story with food to inspire others—and invite them to hear from the Savior as you do. Remember, freedom isn't about perfection. You don't have to "have this down" before you can share your good insight. Sometimes, when I'm in the heart of the mess, I'm better at communicating my hope. Write the names of a few people you can share with—and pray for them today.

Dearest Lord, I don't have to have this all figured out to still be effective in the harvest for souls. Use me where I am today to impact others. Use my brokenness as a door to invite others into Your kingdom love. Amen.

—— DAY 7: REFLECTION AND APPLICATION

Holy Spirit, I love that You bring to remembrance all that Jesus has said and done. Help me to remember my harvest moments. Amen.

On Day Three we talked about protecting our harvest as we studied the concept of hedges. Hedges are a reference to the protective hand of God over our lives and a symbol of how we can pray for specific people and things we ask our Father to shield. Of course, we aren't praying hedges like one would a magical chant, as if a prayer hedge protects from every hard circumstance or inconvenience. On the contrary, we pray a hedge because scripture explains that God places one around us (Job 1), and we join him in his sovereign oversight and care.

In a journal or on the margins of this page, draw circular hedges around the names of people or things you're asking God to protect. As you draw and pray, remember these words of protection from God regarding all that you love. "Protect me as the pupil of your eye; Hide me in the shadow of your wings (Psalm 17:8, CSB).

Lord, I'm protected by You, and I ask for that same protection over those I love. I release all my compulsion and fear to You and know that You are perfect in all Your ways. Amen.

Notes

1.TLB Life Application Bible (Carol Stream, Ill.,: Tyndale House Publishers, 2012), 1007.

2. Spiritual Warfare Bible (Lake Mary, Fla.: Charisma House, 1994), commentary by Ron Phillips, 1274.

WEEK SEVEN: TEACH US TO PRAY

SCRIPTURE MEMORY VERSE
Devote yourselves to prayer, being watchful and thankful. **Colossians 4:2**

I wish I could say I understand prayer. I try to. I really do. But there's so much I still ponder. I sometimes wonder if I'm missing something. Is there a better way that doesn't get distracted, bogged down, or subjected to selfish wanderings? If you've ever felt like this, welcome to the club. I recently asked a large gathering of women how they felt about their prayer life. Most answered, "I'm not sure if I'm doing it right..." while others lamented, "I want to pray but forget or have never really learned how."

The apostle Paul encouraged us to pray without ceasing, and King David seemed to live in a continual stream of prayer as we read the Psalms. Certainly, these leaders wouldn't invite us to it if it weren't possible.   Even Jesus's disciples asked Him to teach them how to pray, which signals that even though they walked, talked, ate, and laughed with Jesus—this was still a confusing concept they fought to understand. I love the words of David as he cried out for deep connection.

> "You, God, are my God,
> earnestly I seek you;
> I thirst for you,
> my whole being longs for you,
> in a dry and parched land
> where there is no water.
> I have seen you in the sanctuary
> and beheld your power and your glory.
> Because your love is better than life,
> my lips will glorify you." (Psalm 63:1-3)

This is the language of prayer. A rich and simple desperation. An open channel to freely express the naked truth surrounding our hearts and our lives. So why is it, at times, foreign or illusive?

I once heard author Francis Chan tell a humorous story about the challenges of prayer. He shared that as much as he wanted to hear wonderful things from God and to converse without ceasing, he found his mind wandering mid-sentence or his heart skipping from topic to topic with no real path or focus. So, to remedy the situation, he built a prayer closet in his garage. The thought was if he had a special place to retreat to, a place with no distractions and a holy purpose to be set apart from the tugs of daily life, surely his mind would concentrate, and his prayer life would soar.

After completing the wooden structure in the back of his garage he entered with anticipation, but shortly after beginning to pray—his mind began to wander once again. "Does my son have plans today after school?" "What do I want to eat for lunch?" All random and unnecessary diversions! He laughed as he said, "The problem wasn't in where I was praying but how I was viewing prayer."

If prayer is communion with God, the unending flow of response to being awakened to his presence, how do we harness it to impact our day-to-day struggles and the nobler issues of praying outward for the world?

As we move towards living *Beyond Free*, prayer is both a healing balm and lightning rod of strength. This week we'll look at how to experience both.

—— DAY 1: PRAYER OF SURRENDER

Jesus, I admit that my prayer life can be scattered. It's not that I don't long to pray deeply, because I do. I ask for maturity in prayer that overcomes my flesh and leads me to communion with You. Amen.

On our journey toward freedom, there's a gem that often gets shoved aside or forgotten. That gem is prayer. As believers we give a lot of lip service to it, but if we're honest, a lot of what we think is prayer is worry, doubt, fear, cynicism, or unbelief—wrapped with pretty-sounding Christian-ese at the beginning and the end.

"Oh, dear Lord ...
Worry, doubt, fear, cynicism, unbelief, repeat over and over...
In Jesus' name...Amen"

One of the keys to overcoming the habits and behaviors we long to overcome is understanding the role prayer plays in the process. If Paul said to pray without ceasing, why isn't it easier?

Please turn to Mark 14:32-38. What were the disciples doing as Jesus was in agony praying?

How long was the timeframe Jesus had been praying and hoped his disciples would have prayed too (vs. 37)?

_____

What reason did Jesus give as to why it's hard to pray (vs. 38)?

_____

_____

Brilliantly, Jesus explained what we struggle so hard to understand when it comes to prayer. "The Spirit is willing, but the flesh is weak." This is why we fall asleep praying—why our minds wander, and we suddenly think about tacos while travailing for someone in need! *Lord help us—our flesh is weak.* But we mustn't throw in the towel and leave it there. We must pursue the deeper facets of faith that Jesus invites us to. Prayer is one of them.

When I began to live *Beyond Free*, one of the first things to change was my prayers. Instead of offering whining prayer like, "Oh Lord, why don't you ever seem to help me with my food issues?" or blaming prayer like, "God, it's your fault! You created me with a big appetite and I can't overcome the way you made me!" I began to offer prayers of surrender. There was a sense of being broken in these prayers—and broken is God's favorite posture for healing power. When we're broken we're not proud, arrogant, or numb. We're surrendered to absolute dependence on God's hope and his will. Broken is not weak. As a matter of fact, broken is strong.

Turn to Philippians 2:8-16. How did Jesus model being broken but not weak in verses 8-11?

_____

_____

Why do you think Paul instructed believers to "work out" their salvation (vs. 12)? What is the outcome of surrendering ourselves to this process (vs. 13)?

_____

_____

Now turn to Philippians 4:4-9. Write verse 6 below.

_____

_____

_____

In a few short verses the Apostle Paul flipped our prayers on their side. Verse 6 lays out the plan for surrendered prayer. I believe the opposite of anxious is surrendered, and Paul wrote, "Do not be anxious about anything, but in every situation, by prayer and petition, with thanksgiving, present your requests to God" (Philippians 4:6). Add the word **surrender** into the following:

Do not be anxious about anything, but _____ in every situation—by prayer and petition, with thanksgiving—presenting your request to God.

What happens when we pray this way (vs.7)?

_____

_____

The prayer of surrender tells God he's in charge. It's not helpless, but rather, filled with trust in the One who can truly change us and change circumstances. The result of surrendered prayer is a mind surrounded by the peace of Jesus.

Re-read verses 8-9. The chart below shows the distinction between things we're told to think on and their opposites. Circle any words you gravitate to when you think about yourself.

What is true...	What is fake, counterfeit, a lie, an accusation
What is noble...	What is shameful, sinful, cheap, pathetic, selfish
What is right...	What is screwy, careless, foolish, compulsive
What is pure...	What is spoiled, false, dishonest, flawed, corrupt
What is lovely...	What is unpleasant, unappealing, ugly, unattractive
What is admirable...	What is worthless, pitiful, imperfect, unlikeable

Some of the antonyms for the words Paul tells us to focus on in Philippians seem harsh. Yet, these are the words many of us use to describe our habits, our bodies, and our outlook when it comes to change.

One of the words that jumped at me is selfish. This word has haunted me for years. After my dad's car wreck when I was nine, things were in such a state of chaos I didn't know what was normal or how to process the bombarding darkness that would, at times, attack my mind. My grandparents were my safety, and during one of my grandmother's extended visits she purchased a doll to take back to one of the children that lived next door to her on the East Coast. I reacted like a young girl might, stating that I, too, would love a doll. We rarely received gifts of this nature, and it seemed normal to ask my grandma for something she was willing to get a neighborhood child.

Mom was in a foul mood (alcohol and depression were her constant companions), and she slapped me with her words. She said I was the most selfish child she'd ever seen, and she continued to use that word against me in the following years. The truth was she battled severe selfishness and narcissism. Hurting people tend to put their greatest shortcomings on those around them, even naming others with the name of their pain. My name became Selfish, and it wasn't until I began to mature in Christ that I realized that was never my name! As a matter of fact, it was a false name that offends the Lord I now serve.

Think about the words you circled on the previous page (or perhaps words that are not on this list but plague you mentally). How did they begin to attach to your life? Can you think of a time or memory when you first began to feel that way? Write the word (s) and explain below.

Today is your day to surrender that word and renounce its power. A Prayer of Surrender is the start to redefining our thought patterns and habitual strains. Start by praying this scripted prayer, then write a personalized Prayer of Surrender of your own.

My Lord, I hand over the rights to my life, and all the poor choices I've ever made. I realize I must be broken to be healed, and my way has not worked. I'm asking for a supernatural touch by You, Jesus—a touch that will reveal my inadequacies, yet not bind me to shame or a sense of hopeless defeat. I renounce any words or names spoken over me that don't reflect Your purpose or the way You have prepared the path of my life. Jesus, You are new life and new hope. The joy of surrender is I don't have to carry the burden of defeat. Surrender is giving over not giving up. I give to You all my thoughts, habits, and behaviors. Create in me a new heart and a new desire to please You in the way I eat and view food. I am forever Yours.

My Prayer of Surrender:

Lord, thank You for the power of surrender. I give You all that I am. Take away any words or names placed on my life that are false. Replace them with Your holy name. Amen.

—— DAY 2: PRAY

Lord, every word and thought from You brings peace. May we be so intimate that healing stirs throughout my body, mind, and spirit—and may healing overflow to others who long for it too. Amen.

Mention the word healing in Christian circles, and you'll get responses swaying from apathy to alarm. Why is healing a catalyst for misunderstanding? Perhaps we're not sure how it's supposed to work, so instead of pressing towards illumination, we run for safety.

In *Prayer: Finding the Heart's True Home*, Richard Foster explains that healing prayer is part of the normal Christian life. He says, "God cares as much about the body as he does the soul, as much about the emotions as he does the spirit. The redemption that is in Jesus is total, involving every aspect of the person—body, soul, will, mind, emotions, spirit."[1]

In First Place for Health we're fully sold out to this thinking, so how do we approach healing prayer with bold faith and common sense? First, we need to remember that God uses both faith and common sense to change us. Faith believes in supernatural help while common sense does what's in front of us. Common sense says "Go to a doctor" when you're sick or "Go to bed" when you're exhausted. It says, "Eat more healthy food and stop when you're full." You get the point. Even Jesus used medical techniques of the ancient world when he performed many of his miracles.

Turn to Mark 7:33-34 and John 9:6. What do both these miracles have in common?

In Jesus's day (and even today) saliva was widely reported to have healing properties.

It was used for boils, snakebites, and eye diseases. No wonder, as the enzymes within saliva have strong antibacterial properties that promote healing. In many healing encounters Jesus was using common sense as well as his supernatural touch to bring change and restore health.

For most of us, common sense prayers are what we're most familiar with. "Lord, give me a desire to eat more vegetables and less processed foods." "Help me to value myself as more than the number I see on the scale." These are wonderful prayers, but we need to go deeper. We need to ask for the supernatural power of God to truly impact our minds, bodies, spirits, and souls. To begin, let's look at things that get in the way of healing prayer.

We pray, and nothing seems to change.

There are many answers. It's important to note that to God, time is not the same as it is to us. To God, time is a tool...to us, it's a measure of delayed and accelerated response. We pray and want immediate results, while to God, sometimes the process is the result. For example, you may want a quick healing when it comes to food, while His intent is healing you through the process of discipline and obedience.

We are in the way of God's next step!

At a speaking event, a young woman came for prayer explaining that she was begging God for her heart's desire. More than anything she wanted to meet a husband she could share her life with, a man who would treasure and value her. I asked if she was seeing anyone and she said, "Well, I'm living with a guy that's a real loser. I'm just staying with him until God brings my real man." Often, this is the way we pray for healing. We're continuing in a harmful behavior while asking God to relieve the pain!

We're in a hurry to see results, and when we don't, we lose faith.

I've prayed for healing in many areas of my life, both physical and emotional. I struggled with debilitating asthma for years. I began to pray for supernatural healing when I was in my twenties. Now, in my fifties, I rarely use an inhaler and have forgotten I ever struggled with it like I did! That's not to say I don't have an inhaler in my purse, because I do. It's just that through time and best practices, asthma no longer defines me or dictates my day. Some healings are instant, and others take time. Usually, Jesus allows us to be a part of the healing by asking us to participate in the prayer in a meaningful way. He may ask us to go, listen, walk, or change direction. If we're in a hurry to see results, we may miss the greater healing Jesus is trying to do.

Do you relate to one of the above? Describe why.

_____

_____

_____

Please turn to John 5:1-9. What strange question did Jesus ask in verse 6?

_____

_____

_____

Scripture says Jesus knew this man had been 38 years in his infirmity, yet he asked a profound question. I believe when it comes to healing prayer, it's the first question Jesus asks. So, let's ask it of ourselves. Do you want to get well? Before you smirk and say, "Of course I do," think of the excuses you put in the way of your healing. List some of your excuses below.

(Here's a few I've used in the past. "I'm too stressed and food is what I look forward to" or "Food is the only vice I have; there are lots of things worse.")

_____

_____

_____

_____

The man by the pool had his excuses too—but note that part of this man's healing was the way he participated in the change. Jesus told him to get up, take what he'd been lying on, and walk. This man's healing was then his story—and his story became his call. Healing prayer was answered as Jesus cut through excuses and gave this man new legs to stand.

Now please turn to Matthew 8:1-4. What did Jesus ask the leper to do after he was healed?

_____

_____

_____

It's beautiful to see that Jesus first touched the leper, which flew in the face of a society that shunned lepers and cast them into isolation. It reminds us that Jesus touches the ugliest parts of our lives willingly and lovingly. After he touched this man and healed him, he told him to go give an offering to the priests. In Jewish culture if people were healed of leprosy (which rarely happened), they had to be examined by a priest to see if they could re-enter society. This was not only demeaning, but in addition to the humiliation, the leper had to pay for the right to be accepted.

In this story I'm reminded that healing prayer is often answered with some required follow-through. Jesus does the healing, but we must follow up on the miracle that he's done. When we think of a healing with food, we often think that one day we magically don't have a desire to overeat and we're instantly in love with Brussels sprouts! When I was healed and set free, I embarked on a lifetime of healthy choices. I was healed of the emotional slavery to food, but still, thirty-five years later, I humbly follow through with what keeps me on track.

To experience healing prayer—let's note the steps to growing in its grasp.

- **Discernment:** We must listen well to ourselves, our bodies, our thought patterns, and others. Read Psalm 119:66 and Proverbs 16:21. Use them as a first step in healing prayer.
- **Ask:** Ask for what we want and invite God in.
- **Believe:** Individually and in your group (or with a trusted prayer partner)—state the fact that you believe God is bigger than any destruction or problem. Faith grows when we exercise belief.
- **Give thanks:** There's power in the posture of gratitude. After praying for healing, we thank God that He has heard us and is already in the process of moving mountains on our behalf.

Jesus, I come to You and ask that You heal me of this burden. If I'm in the way of healing, reveal to me now how I can move, and stretch me beyond anything I could have ever imagined. Amen.

—— DAY 3: THE PRAYER OF AUTHORITY

Jesus, Your power is above every other force on earth. Your authority tears down any fear I harbor. Today, teach me to stand in Your strength. Amen.

I taught school for over fourteen years and then worked as a consultant for Public Education Business Coalition. I used to say I could walk into a classroom anywhere in the country and within five minutes tell who's in charge. You'd be shocked that in countless classrooms it's not the teacher. Typically, it's the loudest, meanest, or sneakiest student because he has grabbed the power. Many teachers leave the profession because they can't figure out how to gain their rightful authority.

Our lives are a lot like that classroom. Somewhere along the way we've lost control and were not sure how to get it back. We know there's a battle for our minds, but the whole thing can seem so overwhelming...and frankly, weird. I've seen people shouting and commanding the demons out of everything from burnt toast to a rude waitress. Yet, scripture is clear: there's more than what meets the eye to most situations. Thankfully, we never see Jesus screaming like a maniac and acting like a fool. He calmly and profusely took authority, and when He did, things changed.

Jesus was brilliant at prayer commands. He commanded—and circumstances changed, demons fled, and people were healed and set free. Richard Foster notes, "This kind of prayer is peppered all through Jesus' ministry. He compelled the wind and the waves to stop, saying, 'Quiet, be still!' He commanded the lepers, 'Be clean.' He touched blind eyes, saying, 'Be opened.' To the paralytic he ordered, 'Get up.' At the grave of his friend Lazarus he commanded, 'Come forth." To demonic spirits he ordered, 'Come out!'"[2]

I love reading these commands, but it's tempting to think "That's great for Jesus... but He is the Son of God...maker of heaven and earth! I can't pray like he can!" Well, let's see what scripture says.

Please turn to Luke 9:1-2. What did Jesus give the disciples?

_____

_____

_____

_____

It's tempting to think that was then, this is now, but nowhere in the Bible does it say this authority has stopped. Watch the progression of authority play out in these verses.

Read Luke 9:6 and 10:9. What did Jesus tell the disciples to do and what did He ask them to say once they'd carried it through?

_____

_____

_____

_____

WEEK SEVEN   TEACH US TO PRAY

Even if we still have some questions as to whether this authority is ours, the next scripture leaves no room for doubt. Read John 14:12. What kind of works does Jesus say we'll do?

_____

_____

_____

_____

It would be ridiculous to think we'll do more important or grander things than Jesus. This verse simply means our works are greater because we are mere humans; sheer faith and trust in the power of God, not ourselves, bring forth good. I'm thrilled we can pray with the authority Jesus has given us, modeling his calm and sane patterns of prayer.

I've preached at large crusades in Uganda, battled with witchdoctors, and slain the enemy in the wildest of ways—but most of the time the prayer of authority is in our everyday, mundane issues of life. In the strength of God, we learn to take authority over our eating habits, our critical tongues, our panic and anxiety, and our bitter or oversensitive reaction to the way people treat us. These are the areas where authority takes courage.

Turn to Matthew 21:21-22. What does Jesus say we should speak to?

_____

_____

Jesus said to speak to the mountain and tell it to move. He didn't say, "Gather a prayer group...journal for twenty minutes...or set a cute spot for quiet time." We must learn to tell the mountains in our life to move, or we'll keep circling around them and never change course.

Read Exodus 14:13-16. What did God say to do when the Israelites are trapped by the sea?

_____

_____

_____

Moses was speaking beautiful words to the people about standing firm and watching the Lord fight. I love Moses because he had to be shaking in his sandals, yet he projected such strength. But God spoke directly into the situation, and instead of thanking Moses for his kind words he said, "You've prayed about this enough...now you need to speak to the sea!" We may never have to move a physical mountain or part the Red Sea, but we do need to move the mountains and seas that keep us from getting to where God is leading.

Mountains and seas can look like all kinds of things—and typically they're no more than obstacles and excuses. (Please know I have great compassion for the mountains and seas of your life. I've spoken to many in my own life, and I'm cheering for you while you learn to speak to yours.)

What kind of mountains have arisen in your life—making change or growth look impossible?

_____

_____

Now, let's learn to speak prayer commands in authority over them. I've made a list of some to get us going.

I want to overeat! I'll try to make good choices tomorrow.
PRAYER COMMAND: Gluttony, leave! You must go...

I'm holding back kindness because I've been hurt.
PRAYER COMMAND: Unforgiveness, flee. You don't represent Christ.

I'm overcome with fear and anxiety. I see no way out of my circumstances.
PRAYER COMMAND: Fear, I reject you. Anxiety, get out. Jesus gives me peace!

Add your own and practice your authority to pray with bold commands.

_____

PRAYER COMMAND:

_____

PRAYER COMMAND:

_____

PRAYER COMMAND:

As we begin to take authority, all kinds of things change. Let's close today by meditating on this verse from the Psalms: "For He spoke, and it was done; He commanded, and it stood fast" Psalm 33: 9 (NASB).

Jesus, You have given me authority to do great things. May my actions and prayer reflect the power You have given me. Amen.

—— DAY 4: PRAY WITHOUT STOPPING!

Lord, I don't want a life of dull prayer—I want to be alive to Your power and presence. Show me how. Amen.

I've always been fascinated by the story of Brother Lawrence. He was a lay brother in a Carmelite monastery in Paris in the 1600s. Although he spent most of his time in the kitchen washing pots and pans, he committed himself to understanding the presence of God in a unique way. His goal was to have God on his mind and in his thoughts at all times. He longed to be in a constant flow of engagement and enjoyment with his Lord.

He shared it took time (almost ten years), but he truly began to live and function in constant communion with God. Just the thought of this is thrilling—but it's also overwhelming. How does one learn to think about and commune with God constantly? The closest I've come was when I first became a believer. For a period of six months, Jesus was on my mind every minute. I'm not kidding. I remember a time period of about five minutes when a moment of worry or distraction came in. I quickly apologized to the Lord and said I hated to not have Him front and center of my thoughts at all times. As the years (and marriage, pro-baseball, babies, jobs, finances, running ministries) crowded in—he has always been my supreme friend and Lord, but my mind has entertained lots of gaps of thinking. The more I've matured and fought battles on the front line for the kingdom, the more I've had to rope in my thoughts and concentrate on His presence. It hasn't been easy. But God never invites us to something He doesn't equip us for. If unceasing prayer and fellowship with God were not possible, He wouldn't ask us to join Him in it.

Please read the following scriptures and jot down what God is asking us to do. 1 Thessalonians 5:17:

Romans 12:12:

Ephesians 6:18:

Colossians 4:2:

There's a pattern in these scriptures that lays out the beauty of possibility. Unceasing prayer is so much more than rote memorization or formulaic routine. It's an ongoing love chat with the God of the universe. Jesus understands this isn't an easy concept to understand.

Read Luke 18:1 and write the verse below.

In our efforts to pray at all times we should not lose heart. But most of our lives look like prayer sprinkles rather than a drenching of prayer. How can we move from a sprinkle to a deluge of prayer in his presence? Oswald Chambers wrote, "If we think of prayer as the breath in our lungs and the blood from our hearts, we think rightly. The blood flows ceaselessly, and the breathing continues ceaselessly; we are not conscious of it, but it is always going on. Prayer is not an exercise, it is the life."[3]

I've found help in my pursuit of a ceaseless prayer life in the notion of breath prayer. This type of prayer has its roots in the Psalms, where a phrase might be repeated over and over to focus the mind on a particular idea. Like the rhythm of breath, these words offer comfort and assurance as we inhale and exhale. King David was a master of breath prayer. Let's study some of the prayers he offered.

Turn to Psalm 23:1. This is a common prayer David offers throughout the Psalms.

What does he pray?

Psalm 46:1. What do the sons of Korah offer as breath prayer here?

Psalm 51:10. What does David cry out to God?

Sometimes it seems as though David is whispering to himself—inviting God into a prayerful tryst that only the two of them understand. Like breathing, the rhythm of this type of prayer redirects and refocuses a wandering mind or heart that needs to be reassured.

Richard Foster guides us into discovering breath prayer for ourselves:

- Sit in silence, being held in God's presence.
- Allow God to call you by name.
- Allow God to ask you, "What do you want?" "What is stirring within?"
- Perhaps a single word or phrase will surface—peace, faith, courage—"to understand your truth" or "to be free from harm."
- Connect your word or phrase to a comfortable way you express your praise to God—Savior, Abba, Sweet Lord, my Father.
- Say the prayer within the confines of one breath.4

My recent breath prayer revolves around justice being served in a volatile situation. I've found myself studying scripture on God as a good Judge. Here's my current breath prayer:

My righteous Judge...you fight my battles.

Using the steps given, create your own breath prayer. Write it below.

Pray this prayer throughout the day as you train your mind to allow God to dominate as many minutes as possible while you're awake. To "pray without ceasing" is our goal.

Dearest Lord, my aim is to never stop communicating throughout the day. As I sort through my thoughts, Holy Spirit, remind me to pray rather than wander. Amen.

—— DAY 5: CONTINUE TO SERVE

Jesus, I pray for an increase of influence and favor. May I boldly take new ground for You. Amen.

Several years ago a two-sentence prayer took the country by storm. Tucked in some obscure verses in 1 Chronicles, a man named Jabez was singled out for the way he prayed. When Dr. Bruce Wilkinson wrote the book *The Prayer of Jabez*, he had no idea he was stoking the fire of millions of people ready to blaze with confidence in prayer. These two verses in scripture launched a movement. Let's go to these verses and try to understand why.

Turn to 1 Chronicles 4:9-10. How did Jabez get his name?

The first thing to note is his mother was a bit shocked by his birth. The name *Jabez* literally means "distress." This is a good reminder for those of us who came into the world unwanted or with hardship. God has plans for our lives we can't see. I believe his mama eventually wished she hadn't given her son such a harsh name because as Jabez grew, he was more honorable and distinguished than his brothers.

What does verse 10 say Jabez was known for?

Unlike many Bible heroes known for action, Jabez was simply known for prayer. His short but powerful prayer model concentrates on four areas: **blessing, influence, presence and protection.**

What's the first thing Jabez asked God to do?

It might seem self-centered to ask God for blessing, but it's a brilliant thing to do. We need more blessing to be better equipped to make a difference for the kingdom.

Turn to James 4:2-3. What's the problem with the way we sometimes ask?

It's important to understand that God longs to bless us, but He wants us to come to Him with the right kind of heart. Let's frame this within our struggles with food. Let's say we ask God to bless us and help us lose weight. This is an okay request but not a fully mature one. If we asked God to help us be free from this struggle and to lose and maintain a good weight so we could invite others into the freedom and hope they can find in God—that's a real blessing God longs to give. It's centered on kingdom purpose rather than "me" purpose. When we ask for blessing with the motivation to not only help ourselves, but also help others, that gets his attention.[5]
Pray this prayer of blessing:

> *Father, I pray that You would bless me with more than I need so that I can bless others. I pray for wisdom, discernment, and provision, so I can generously give both physically and spiritually. I ask that You give me greater spiritual gifting so I can strengthen Your people and be more effective for Your kingdom. Help me keep your blessings in perspective, so I never become self-serving but stay focused on using what You have given me to serve other people. Amen.*

After blessing, what's the next thing Jabez asked God to do?

This is the request that excites me. Every morning before getting out of bed, Bobby and I pray this prayer, and I repeat this line twice because it means that much to me: "enlarge my territory." Some versions use the word borders, but I like territory because it seems so vast. Each of us is given a territory to influence, conquer, and maintain. That territory can include our families, work opportunities, ministry, relationships, health, influence within the community, position, or favor in our realm of expertise or passion. When we ask God to expand this territory, we're asking Him to push the boundaries out and give us more than we dreamed. So often, we're content with a little patch of territory rather than asking God to expand what we have! I never dreamed I'd be speaking around the world and running a place in Uganda. I've written several books and a TV show—and gratefully and humbly...I'm just getting started.

What are some of the areas you'd like to see God push your borders or expand your territory? Please take this seriously as limiting your borders hurts not only you but also those you could potentially impact.

After expanding his territory, what are the final two things Jabez requested of God? (1 Chronicles: 10)

In scripture God's hands are mentioned repeatedly as a sign of power and protection. Read the following scriptures and note the power of God's hands:

Psalm 16:11:

Luke 23:46:

Mark 14:62

Isaiah 40:11-12

The hands of God represent his presence and position. Remember that Jesus is seated at the right hand of God. Jabez understood that when God placed His hand on him, it meant His attention and presence was upon him. We, too, can ask for God's hands to hold us, protect us, teach us, and guide us.

Finally, when we're blessed, taking new territory, and thriving in God's presence, the enemy will rear his head. This is why Jabez asked to be kept from harm or pain. Jesus has already won the victory, so we don't need to fear the enemy. Jabez wisely asked God to be kept from harm...and so should we.

I love the final sentence in this scripture, "And God granted his request" (1 Chronicles 4:10). The whole thing is so simple and clear. Although life can feel anything but simple, we need to remember this concise and faithful prayer sums up the essence of our hope.

Jesus, like Jabez, I pray for Your favor and protection. I love the borders and territory that You are expanding in my life. Help me to bravely ask for more. Amen.

—— DAY 6: REFLECTION AND APPLICATION

Lord, prayer is my communion with You. May I partake often and with an open heart. Amen

This week we covered a lot of ground in our study of prayer. We focused on prayers of surrender, healing, and authority—as well as learning to pray without ceasing and for territory and blessing. On a separate piece of paper or in a journal, select one of the types of prayer we've covered and make it your own. Share with God the questions you have or the excitement you feel towards unlocking a new treasure in communicating with Him. Then use the following prompts to apply what you've learned about this type of prayer.

- As I pray I long to focus on _____.
- I'm free to explore this new concept or go deeper with a concept I've known but haven't practiced.
- Lord, I hand over skepticism or doubt as I move into a deeper prayer life with You.
- I will apply this new type of prayer to my eating habits and desire for weight loss in the following ways:

_____

After completing this, consider sharing your thoughts with your prayer partner and listening to hers or his. Commit to praying for one another's new prayer focus.

Holy Spirit, I ask for fresh revelation as to how to pray. Take me to new places as I journey with You. Amen

—— DAY 7: REFLECTION AND APPLICATION

Jesus, my day is in Your capable hands. I rest in the presence of Your smile. Amen.

On Day Four we went through the steps of crafting our own breath prayer. King David had many breath prayers that stand out as phrases we're familiar with today. "The Lord is my shepherd" is the most famous breath prayer he uttered, but many others resonate as we read the Psalms. Typically, if he repeated a phrase or concept later in the Psalm, this was his breath prayer. Read the following Psalms and note the breath prayer that swells from these verses.

Psalm 57:1 _____

Psalm 42:1 _____

Psalm 27:14 _____

Psalm 18:1-2 _____

Write the breath prayer you crafted on Day Four below and repeat it throughout the day as a private offering between you and God.

MY BREATH PRAYER

_____

_____

Notes

1. Richard Foster, Prayer: Finding the Heart's True Home (San Francisco: HarperCollins, 1992), 203.

2. Foster, Prayer, 234.

3. Oswald Chambers, My Utmost for His Highest (Ulrichsville, Ohio: Barbour, 2000), 105.

4. Adapted from my book Spirit Hunger (Grand Rapids, Mich.: Zondervan, 2012), 80-81.

5. Thanks to the Hope City Church Prayer Manual for guidance on the Prayer of Jabez.

WEEK EIGHT: GOD ON THE MOVE

SCRIPTURE MEMORY VERSE
Do you not know that in a race all the runners run, but only one gets the prize? Run in such a way to get the prize. 1 Corinthians 9:24

Growing up, we spent hours outside. We'd play long games of hide-and-go-seek and kickball—then we'd jump on our bikes and pretend to be racecar drivers. When we tired of that, we'd tumble on the grass doing cartwheels and handstands. Never once did we measure or dread our activity. It was a natural state of movement and enjoyment. Why, when we become adults, do things shift? Why does being active take real planning and exercise seem like a chore?

The world has changed. Most of us are not farmers or livestock wranglers. We don't hunt or fish for our next meal, and we drive from place to place rather than walk. We've gotten larger and more sedentary—but still, our bodies are designed to move! In the motion of busy days and endless demands, we must find ways to be active and alive. I can't think of one person I love in the Bible that was a couch potato...not one.

Moses was a shepherd who could hike mountains, even in his old age. Peter, Andrew, James, and John were brawny fisherman with muscular arms—used to casting nets and pulling in loads of fish. Elijah was a runner who outran a king's transportation from Mount Carmel back to town. Even Jesus and the disciples walked miles daily as they ministered from town to town, region to region. Imagine what would've happened if they had quit because they were out of shape or didn't feel like moving to a new, distant place. "I'm too exhausted to get out and walk!" "I don't feel I like it...my legs hurt." "Pass me some more bread and wine...I'm staying put today!"

I love a scripture tucked away in the third letter of John. He was writing to a beloved friend and believer named Gaius, and opened his letter with this: "Dear Friend, I am praying that all is well with you and that your body is as healthy as I know your soul is" (1 John 1:2, TLB). John was concerned with his friend's spiritual **and** physical well-being. Some Christians today think caring about our bodies is silly, while others compulsively obsess over every inch of body fat and jiggle.

It's important to remember that God cares about both our bodies and our souls. Both neglecting our bodies and our health and overindulging our fleshly appetites are misguided. We need to discipline and move our bodies, so we're our best for God's service.

—— DAY 1: DOES GOD WEAR A FITBIT?

Father, I know that to have good friends, I need to be one. Show me how to be an encourager. Amen.

Our title today may sound ridiculous, but I can't help but wonder how God views our attempts to be fit. Once, while sitting in my dirty office in the run-down building we rented in Uganda (before building our own), a woman from the United States came to visit us with her father who lived in the capital city of Uganda. I'd met the woman on a flight to Baltimore. She explained that after leaving Uganda as a college student and making a life in the U.S., she was planning to return home to Africa soon to visit her family. She promised to come see us at The Vine if our schedules ever crossed paths. I was shocked when she followed through. So, there we were, the three of us, her elderly father leaning against the stained wall, when suddenly an alarm on her wrist went off! It was her Fitbit signaling she'd been sitting too long, and it was time to move. Her father shook his head in bewilderment. He looked at me and asked, "How can my daughter, who was raised here in Uganda, be concerned with eating too much? And why does she need a watch to tell her to move?" He had a point. How strange it must have seemed to a man who'd spent his life making sure his family had enough to eat; moving was as natural as breathing for him.

I'm not criticizing any apparatus that helps us be active. On the contrary, I'm just fascinated with the effort it takes. In my own life I have to pre-plan and schedule it. I'm one of those rare people who love to work out. I slap on my headphones and sing worship music so loud the people sweating around me think I'm nuts. But, I'm embarrassed to say there are countless times I'm in the parking lot of the gym answering work emails or calls and never actually make it in the door.

Ultimately, it comes down to the why behind the what. Why do we work out and for what reward? What motivates me more than having thin thighs or buttoning jeans easily is the fact that God was active and on the move. Anything he does I want to model.

Turn to Genesis1:2. What does the Bible say God's spirit was doing?

Some translations say God was hovering and others say he was moving. Either way, he was active.

Now read the rest of the creation story from Genesis 1:3 thru 2:2. What did God need to do on the seventh day?

Can you imagine the energy it took to create everything we know as the heavens and earth? It was so physical and active that God took a rest on the seventh day—not because he was lazy or exhausted, but because this creation activity was good—and the day of rest was holy. The beauty of resting comes from the activity it took to need the rest. Some of us are not active enough to ever need rest. We're invited to something much more rewarding.

Turn to 1 Corinthians 9:24-27. Write verse 26 below.

In these verses Paul used the example of a race to describe our need for self-discipline. Some would argue this is only to be spiritually fit, but I think his meaning was deeper. Paul said we don't run aimlessly or box at the air and used two very physical activities to make a point about being intentional with movement. He did not say if we run or box (or stay active in some sense) but when we do—we do it with intention, not in aimless pursuit. Aimless pursuit is starting to walk and stopping after a few short days or sitting in the gym parking lot instead of going in or putting on your workout clothes and crawling back into bed. You get the point.
In verse 27 what did Paul explain?

Paul pressed in further by saying, "No, I strike a blow to my body and make it my slave...." (1 Corinthians 9:27). So often, we let our bodies dictate what we do rather than use sound discipline. If our body feels lazy, we let it languish. If we want to overeat, we succumb to the desire. Paul ended the thought by saying, "...after I have preached to others, I myself will not be disqualified for the prize" (1 Corinthians 9:27). In other words, if I expect other people to have it together and live right lives, I had better do the same. When it comes to being active or fit, we don't have to compete with anyone else or try to fit into the mold of what works for them. If walking around the block several times is the best you can do—do it with intention. If you're struggling to get outdoors or had a recent injury, chair and floor workouts are good too. As long as we make choices to be fit and truly try, we're not disqualified.

At this point, if we're still tempted to make excuses, the next scripture is convincing. Turn to Luke 1:5-40. Although we're very familiar with this story, try to read it from a fresh perspective. What did Gabriel share with Mary in verses 36-37?

Notice what Mary's first reaction was when she heard the impossible news from the angel. She quickly left to visit her relative Elizabeth in the hill country of Judea. I want you to understand the full gravity of this verse. It was a ninety-mile walk to the village of Ein Karem, Elizabeth's home. Mary traveled alone (perhaps in a caravan but without anyone she knew) and was on foot. Only wealthy people had access to donkeys and animals for travel, and to top it off, she may have been feeling a bit of nausea from being newly pregnant. If she walked three miles an hour, it would have taken Mary more than thirty hours to get to Elizabeth—and she got there in a hurry.

She and Elizabeth shared three beautiful months together, and then Mary did the trek home again. Friends, if the pregnant mother of God can offer a walk like this to be where she needed to be, how much more can we offer?

Jesus, help me to do what it takes to be who I need to be inside this body. You've given it to me, and I choose to honor you within it. Amen.

—— DAY 2: REBUILD OUR TEMPLE

Lord, just as You instructed Your people to rebuild Your temple, we ask You to help us rebuild ours. Our bodies are the temple in which You dwell. Amen.

In the Old Testament God talked a lot about temples. He constantly instructed the Jews as to how temples should be built and what should happen within them. I've always thought, "That's nice, but it doesn't really apply to me now." It wasn't until I made the connection between the Old Testament temple and my New Testament body that the whole thing made sense. The temple is one of the fascinating symbols the Holy Spirit uses to get our attention.

Please turn to 2 Corinthians 6:16-18. What did Paul call us?

Just as there were requirements to make things clean in the temple before the living God, so we are to separate ourselves and be clean from the stains of sin as God our Father beautifully loves us.

Now turn to 1 Corinthians 3:16-17. How did Paul describe our temple?

Now, before you feel overwhelmed with a rundown or out-of-shape temple, let's watch an inspiring temple story unfold.

Please turn to Haggai and read chapter 1. What does the prophet say we must do in verse 5?

The prophet said we must consider our ways. He then explained how we sow but reap no harvest. We are never satisfied with our food and drink, and our clothes don't keep us warm.

What did Haggai instruct in verses 7-8?

Haggai gave a solution to the empty pursuit the Jews were struggling to understand— rebuild my temple and I will be pleased. Because the people had not given God first place in their lives, their material possessions did not satisfy. Their attempts to sow and reap did not produce fruit because the temple was in ruins—and their time was spent on things that didn't please God! The good news is the people began rebuilding the temple just twenty-three days after Haggai preached this message. The people were quick to see the problem and work towards the solution. Often, we hear good messages or read good Bible studies, but never truly change. Haggai said to "Go up into the mountains and bring down timber..." (vs. 8). This was going to be physical work and effort, but God would be pleased.

How can we begin to rebuild our temples today? No delay. What steps can we take to make exercise and healthy eating a reality not just a dream?

_____

_____

_____

What message did the Lord give to the people in verse 13? Write it below.

_____

_____

_____

Zerubbabel was the governor of Judah during Haggai's time. He demonstrated courage both to move forward with God...and to wait. Work had begun on the temple years before, but after some skirmishes with hostile neighbors, the work was halted. For 16 years the temple went untouched, while what began as a good work laid in ruins. At just the right time Haggai and later the prophet Zechariah encouraged Zerubbabel it was time to start again...and this time, success!

Read Haggai 2. What encouragement did God give Zerubbabel in verse 23?

_____

_____

_____

Most people have tried to overcome what hurts them. Overeaters diet...compulsive drinkers quit for periods of time... and people who attract bad company try to make new friends. We've all tried and failed at something, but God has fresh words for fresh resolve. This time things will change. Freedom is real, and the truth does set you free. God gives you the same encouragement He gave Zerubbabel: he has chosen you to overthrow whatever has kept you down.

Lord Jesus, thank You for Your encouragement and the power to rebuild my temple. I know it takes work, but I have the courage You give me. You are with me, and You are enough. Amen.

—— DAY 3: CHANGE IS MORE THAN WISHFUL THINKING
Jesus, I'm so excited to do things Your way. You give fresh hope when I'm stale and worn out. I give You my resolve and ask for your supernatural breath. Amen.

It's hard to change the habits we've formed over years—but loving Jesus is all about change. If we're not changing, there's a good chance we're judging, doubting, criticizing, or envying those who are. The Bible is clear: God is a God of hope and faith ushers in the impossible. Over the course of my life, I've changed physically and emotionally more than you can imagine.

Physically, I was the girl who grew up on Captain Crunch, canned chili, and cookie dough. No joke. I don't remember ever eating fresh fruit or vegetables unless it was a banana surrounded by ice cream and syrup. When I started to get free, I asked God to change my taste buds. Why not? If He could part the sea and make the sun stand still, how are little buds on a tongue a challenge? The more I ate carrots, the less I craved candy. Now, roasted veggies with sea salt rival any food you could put before me. That's change.

Emotionally, I begged God to give me a man who would never cheat, children who would never be harmed, and stability to stay somewhere and plant roots. Instead, my marriage went through the wringer but is stronger than ever, two of my three kids were harmed in horrendous ways but have emerged mightily, and we've moved nearly fifty times in our life in professional baseball. However, planted roots can leave flowering growth over a large territory, not a small plot. That's change.

Please turn to 1 Corinthians 15:58. What does God instruct us to do?

Paul said we must give ourselves fully to the work of the Lord. I used to think that was just holy work, like sharing the Gospel and helping the poor. Now I know different. It's just as holy to go walk as it is to serve. Both require obedience, and both have reward.

Now turn to 1 Corinthians 15:37-44. What did Paul mention in verse 38?

This chunk of scripture is both strange and refreshing. On one hand he talked about our earthly bodies, and on the other, our bodies in heaven. To begin, he compared our bodies to a seed that's planted. Paul wrote,

"When you put a seed into the ground it doesn't grow unless it 'dies' first. And when the green shoot comes up out of the seed, it is very different from the seed you first planted. For all you put into the ground is a dry little seed of wheat or whatever it is you are planting, then God gives it a beautiful new body—just the kind he wants it to have; a different kind of plant grows from each kind of seed." (1 Cor. 15: 36-38, TLB)

We know our bodies will be different in heaven than they are on earth, but this image is for the body we're living in now as well. Paul used the seed image to show that after being planted, the seed appears to die but actually is experiencing new life. Some of us need to host a funeral for our old ways. A eulogy needs to be given for our old body and the habits that have gotten it to the weight or shape it is now. When old ways die, new bodies happen.

What would a perfect body look like to you? Take some time with this. Your answer may surprise you.

_____

_____

_____

Scripture assures that someday we'll have new and perfect bodies. One commentary notes our bodies will still have our personalities. I just hope mine won't have my current abs! The problem is we live inside the body we have now, flawed and at times weak—yet mighty in purpose. During our time on earth it's our job to take good care of our body and treat it with care. The process of change is a wise balance of courage and tenacity. We ask God for new victories and listen to his strategies to win.

When David was getting settled as King of Israel an old enemy raised its head—the Philistines. Hadn't he already defeated their big giant Goliath? Hadn't he already had victory in this area that sparked change in the confidence and history of a nation? Yes. But this was a battle he'd have to keep growing with. It wasn't once and done, and neither is our battle for change.

Turn to 1 Chronicles 14:8-17. How many times in these verses did the enemy attack? What did David do before battle?

_____

You'd think after defeating his foe once it'd be over. After all, God gave the strategy. Shouldn't it be final? Yet, soon after the victory the nasty enemy was prowling again. The second time David inquired God gave a different plan of attack. A sound from the top of the poplar trees meant God was before them.

To me, what's interesting is that after the first victory in Baal-Perazim, David might have gotten lax and forgotten to stay strong and committed to battle. Baal-Perazim means "The Place of Breaking Through" and for many of us, after an initial break-through (weight loss, altered appetites, loose clothing), we let down our guard and settle right back into the patterns we were in before the battle. Verse 12 says the Jews picked up many of the idols left by the Philistines, and David ordered them to be burned. Good for him. But immediately following that, the enemy was back for another round. Wisely, David again asked God for the right strategy, and God gave him something completely new and fresh.

Friends, when it comes to change, we can't assume that God's way of working things out will always be the same. If you seek God's leading as circumstances change, you will not see change as a threat or something you'll fail at—but as an opportunity to see God work in new ways. Some of us have been using the same tools for years with little result. Perhaps years ago you saw results using that strategy, but now you don't. Here are steps toward a new plan:

- Ask God for His guidance, protection, and clarity.
- Assess what tools/strategies worked in the past, and be honest about how they are working today. (Are you stuck with the same workout routine, food choices, or tracking system delivering small or no results?)
- Go to battle with fresh commitment and intrigue. Ask God to give you fresh ideas and new tools that awaken you. You WILL be successful with God and tenacious faith.
- Thank God for success, and turn it into a chance for God's fame to grow. David's fame grew after victory, and he was quick to give the glory back to God. Perhaps God might have you lead a group, speak publicly about your life change, or share your progress in a way others can be inspired and encouraged. The more we change, the more others are invited to believe they can too.

Father, it's incredible to see Your victory strategies. When we feel as though change is impossible, You bring peace and new hope to life. Amen.

—— DAY 4: POWER PERFECTED

Lord God, so many things you teach in the Word need deep revelation and thought. Teach me about true power. Amen

Being married to a pro-athlete and coach, I have seen my share of power. I've watched scrawny men knock a baseball clear out of a ballpark and onto the streets behind a stadium. I've also witnessed power in the hands of politicians when I interned on Capitol Hill and in the elders of a village in Uganda. I've seen power loosed from the tongues of teachers and moms and business leaders—wielding the gavel of decisions that change the course of lives breathlessly waiting to be shaped.

Of all the shapes and forms of power I've witnessed, never have I considered the weak to be strong—or power perfected by weakness. Quite the opposite. It seems power begets power. The stronger people are, the more confidence they have in their power. The apostle Paul presented a radically new and different interpretation of the word power in his letter to the Corinthian church.

Please turn to 2 Corinthians 12:7-10. How did Paul describe power in these verses?

Paul boldly proclaimed things that don't make sense. Power is perfected in weakness? When I am weak I am strong? In the natural world these words war against each other, but in the Spirit, they tame and refine. To understand why Paul penned these words, let's go back and read what led him to this point.

Please read 2 Corinthians 12:1-6. How would you describe what Paul experienced?

Although this is a bit hard to understand, we know that 14 years earlier Paul had some kind of experience that included a glimpse of heaven. Even he wasn't sure if this experience were in his actual body or in a vision, but he shared it to let people know he'd had a unique experience—one so great that he may have been tempted to have been boastful about it. In the aftermath a physical affliction began to surface and proved to stay with him for a while. Some think it was malaria, epilepsy, or some kind of eye disease—whatever the case, it kept him on his knees. It was in this state he proclaimed, "Power is perfected in weakness" and "when I am weak I am strong."

The relevance of focusing on these statements in a chapter centered on fitness is clear. It's weakness that helps us understand the power of being strong. Power is perfected as we trust God daily to shape our weak bodies into something that showcases His strength.

Author Lysa Terquerst shares how she began running. In the beginning she ran in her neighborhood from mailbox to mailbox...then she'd cry. But as she continued to show up for those morning running sessions, God began to perfect her weakness, and now she runs four miles a day. Weak became strong—but first there were some tears. Lysa prepared to exercise with intention. She asked God to make her strong and then she ran with expectation—knowing that God was perfecting her power.

Asthma kept me from running as a child, so when the idea struck me to run as an adult, I was a bit surprised. I couldn't afford a gym membership, and I wanted to push myself to try something new, so I got some running shoes and determined to learn how to run. At first, it felt like my chest might burst and scatter over my Nikes and slick new athletic pants. I could dress the part—but following through with the activity proved to be much harder. I started by walking on a path I loved and periodically running a small portion. I'd add running portions to the walk each day, and before I knew it, I was running the whole route. Now, after years of walking due to some nagging injuries, I've recently begun adding some running sprints into my routine. My muscles are sore, but that's a sign I'm working hard and mixing it up. If we're willing to try—to take on hard new things physically—God supplies the time and endurance for the rest.

One of the most profound scriptures on power is in the book of Isaiah. Please turn to Isaiah 40:28-31. Let's look at these verses bit by bit.

What does verse 28 say about God's character and understanding?

God never gets tired or worn down. His energy level is always 100 percent and his strength is always at maximum.

Write verse 29 on the lines below.

This is the key to increasing power both in our bodies and in our spirits. He increases the power of the weak. What are some ways you need Him to increase your physical power and strength? Be specific.

Verse 31 says those who hope in the Lord will renew their strength and soar on wings like eagles. This verse is rich with meaning. An eagle has the ability to soar. We spend so much energy flapping (trying this and that with no real reward) while the eagle waits for the wind. A wind thermal is a current of air that rises from the atmosphere and will carry an eagle that enters it just right to heights without wasted expended energy. In scripture one of the symbols of the Holy Spirit is wind. How can you soar rather than flap when it comes to fitness? In How can you rely on his thermal power to lift you to new hope and strength?

Finally, verse 31 says we will run and not grow weary, and we will walk and not be faint. For those who feel both weary and faint, remember—it starts from mailbox to mailbox and ends with miles of praise. The point is to start. You can't soar if you don't get up and start. And once you start, keep pushing yourself to soar higher and longer.

Lord, engrave in my mind the image of an eagle soaring. It's a beautiful reminder that I don't have to spend needless energy--but learn to flow in Your currents and the rhythm of Your grace.

—— DAY 5: BE STRONG! EVEN WHEN YOU FEEL WEAK

Lord Jesus, I long to change, and live my life in a body I'm proud of. Cover me during the times I feel weak. Encourage me in the ways of strength. Amen.

It's amazing how small advertising statements can stay with us for years. According to one advertising agency, here are some of the top ten jingles of all time:

- McDonalds: "I'm Lovin It"
- Kit Kat: "Give Me a Break"
- Oscar Mayer: "I Wish I Were an Oscar Mayer Wiener"
- State Farm: "Like a Good Neighbor"
- Alka Seltzer: "Plop, Plop, Fizz, Fizz"

I can recite every single one of these verses and even picture what the people singing them looked like! There's truly power in repetition and something catchy that makes a point. The apostle Paul was especially good at it. And although he wouldn't have called them jingles—many of his phrases stick with me like a commercial ringing in my head.

When Paul wrote to young Timothy, he was pouring out everything he could into a man he considered a son. He was trying to mentor and teach what he knew to this willing new leader before Paul passed on to glory. In his second letter to Timothy, there's a section that has a true jingle. As a matter of fact, it's the subheading in many translations to this chapter of scripture. It simply says...Be Strong!

Please turn to 2 Timothy 2:1-13. What does Paul instruct in verses 1-2?

Paul not only said to be strong, but also commanded us to give the wisdom we learn from his words to other people who will be able to share and teach them as well. This is the power of meeting in a group or sharing your struggles and growth with others. Imagine what your First Place for Health group can be as you begin to authentically live strong together. When we share this new hope with others, strength spreads. Imagine the power of this strength: *I ran a mile today...I walked for 30 minutes...I controlled my appetite and then put on my sneakers and worked out.*

R

ead verse 3. What kind of hardship do you think Paul is referring to? What hardships do you face as you try to live out the gospel and freedom in a real way?

_____

_____

_____

Next, Paul used three examples to highlight his words on strength and overcoming hardships.

The Good Soldier (vs. 3-4): What did Paul say a soldier should do and not do?

_____

_____

_____

One translation says the soldier shouldn't get entangled in the affairs of everyday life but should rise above them to please the one who enlisted him as a soldier. How do we find ourselves entangled in the everyday issues of life rather than rising above them (eating on the run, grabbing handfuls of things we don't even want to eat, putting off exercise or anything that feels hard)?

_____

_____

_____

A Competitive Athlete (vs. 5): What is the only way an athlete can win a prize?

_____

_____

_____

To win, an athlete must follow the rules, and the same goes for us as we try to overcome habits and change. I talk to so many people who think this whole messy weight issue should be an easy fix. Why does it demand so much? Why can't we just pray and instantly be healed? We must learn to follow the rules, and for those of us who like to break them or simply detour daintily around them...this is a deal breaker. Our bodies are built with certain rules attached such as "too much food in, too many pounds on" or "with no or little movement the body breaks down or stubbornly stays fat." It's that simple. God made the rules.

Have you been trying to break or bend the rules while enjoying little or no success? Explain.

A Hardworking Farmer (vs. 6): What can this farmer enjoy when he gives his all?

Here's the joy in all the rules and the hard work: when we do it, we get to enjoy the rewards of it. Guaranteed. Do you remember where Paul was preaching from? A prison, where he says he was "chained like a criminal." But God's word is not chained.

To close our time today, I'd like to share a story with you that's left an edible mark on me. In his book *Every Body Matters*, author Gary Thomas describes a vision he had after a long week of work.[1] He was worn out and discouraged, wondering if his efforts at writing, speaking, and serving the Lord were bearing any fruit. Not one prone to visions, he was a bit surprised at how real this seemed. He pictured himself running along a mountain pass. It was cold and rainy—and the sky was dark with wind. As he ran, he found himself at a wood cabin and was welcomed in by Jesus. He was bloody, sore, and tired—wet from head to toe. Jesus invited him to sit in a chair, and He gave Gary something warm to eat and drink. Then, Jesus removed his soaked shoes, socks, and running clothes—replacing them with dry, sturdy new ones. He gently bandaged the bloody scrapes and wounds that came from running so hard and so long. Then, before walking him to the door He spoke words too precious to share.

As Jesus opened the door of the cabin the winds howled, and the rain came down, but Gary was filled with new life. Jesus kindly placed his hand on Gary's back and said, "Now, Gary, keep running." Perhaps you, like Gary, need a personal touch from Jesus. A tailor-made commission that helps you stay strong in the midst of defeat or discouragement or stay strong as you continue to obey in a quiet and resilient strength. Let's end today in a time of heart-felt prayer.

Dear Jesus, I need a touch from you. I'm weary of trying to "do" right when I simply want to "be" right with you. I need your hands to wash my sores and bandage my wounds—some inflicted by careless people and some inflicted by my own neglectful ways. You say to be strong, and you never tell me to be something you don't help me to become. Today I chose strength because in my weakness You ride in like a champion with powerful resolve. I am strong in the power of Your might. I forever choose You. Amen.

—— DAY 6: REFLECTION AND APPLICATION

Jesus, I know You are taking me to new heights of maturity and grace. I welcome all the ways You teach me. Amen.

On Day Four we talked about the words Paul uttered when faced with challenges: power is perfected in weakness. I thought I understood these words but came to realize my understanding was shallow until a few years back.

I'd been asked to speak at a crusade in Uganda, so I assembled a team of courageous but unprepared middle-aged women to come and serve in a variety of capacities. (For the record, we had an eighteen-year-old and a young woman in her twenties too.) I should have known we were in for a ride when my backpack, filled with my passport and money, was accidentally left on my porch by the sweet girl who loaded our van. I had to send my entire team one day ahead of me   --and only one of them had ever been to Uganda before. When I arrived, it was a sheer miracle I found the little driver who would take me five hours away from the airport into the town we were to work in before going to the crusade.

After three nights of virtually no sleep due to the travel, I accidentally dozed off in my hotel before going to preach my first scheduled day in Uganda. It was late at night before I caught a glimpse of my face in the mirror, and I was appalled at what I saw. In my quick doze early in the morning, a spider marched across my face, biting me upwards of twenty-one times! I looked like an adult with the measles!

To make matters worse, when we arrived at the remote city where the crusade was held, the local pastors hosted a dinner of local food for our team to enjoy. Not wanting to be rude, I ate a little of everything presented and found myself violently ill from midnight on. As I lay writhing in pain, one scripture kept ringing in my ears: power is perfected in weakness. We had traveled across the world and this region was expecting a crusade. They had prepared for almost a year to make it happen. I simply couldn't be sick.

As dawn rolled around I crawled to the shower and somehow stood to wash my hair and body. I put on a dress while barely being able to breathe. My breath prayer was "Power is perfected in weakness...power is perfected in weakness...."

That day I preached three times, and as I looked out over the vast cornfields filled with people, children hanging from the trees to hear the word of God, and those lined up who could never see a doctor but came believing in the power of prayer—I understood Paul's words for the first time. God's power is perfected in our weakness.

Today, reflect on this scripture. His power is connected to your weakness. Instead of fighting it, lean into it.

My Lord, I lean into Your strength to reshape my weakness. I don't have the answers, only the will to surrender. Amen.

—— DAY 7: REFLECTION AND APPLICATION

Dear Holy Spirit, bring new things to my mind. Show me how to view my body and movement in a fresh new way. Amen.

Over the past two weeks we've studied the power of prayer as well as the need to move our bodies. The two can be beautifully woven if we take the time to prepare. When I work out, I have worship music circulating in my head, which always makes the minutes sweeter and more powerful. But the past few years I've tried another new strategy. I bought an index card spiral rolodex that fits in my hands. On the colorful cards I placed a variety of scriptures, inspirational quotes from my favorite author Oswald Chambers, and breath prayers from various seasons of life. No matter how I feel when I begin (tired, discouraged, lacking confidence), by the time I'm done, I feel fired up and ready to go.

Today, reflect on what might focus your mind in a positive way as you move your body for God. Then, not only does your body benefit, but your spirit soars as well.

Jesus, when I dedicate intentional time to moving my body and growing strong in you, everything in my life changes. My body, mind, and spirit are renewed in a personal revival. Amen.

Notes

1. Gary Thomas, Every Body Matters (Grand Rapids, Mich.: Zondervan, 2011), 206-207.

WEEK NINE: WHAT'S GOING ON?

SCRIPTURE MEMORY VERSE
No discipline seems pleasant at the time, but painful. Later on, however, it produces a harvest of righteousness and peace for those who have been trained by it. Hebrews 12:11

Have you ever lived through a timeframe that left you scratching your head in confusion? A time when nothing made sense, and your ability to reason or think rationally seemed to fly out the window? If you've ever wondered "What's going on?" you're in good company. What most of us fail to realize is there are three systems at work in us spiritually. Once we recognize which system is operating, we're much quicker to respond appropriately.

We all face times of disciplining, sifting, and pruning. These are the Biblical systems at work, designed to help us mature and grow. Most people recognize them as hard times—and fail to glean what they're meant to teach.

Disciplining occurs from God our Father when we fail to live by the standards of holiness or protection he's designed in the Bible. He gently but firmly helps us get back on track. Sifting comes from Satan. He has asked permission to shake us up and will try to push us around until we break or fall. Pruning comes from the hand of the Father and occurs because we're doing something right! In this case, God wants our right living to bear more fruit, and pruning is the method He uses to bring it about. All three delicate systems can lead to mature growth if we learn from them. What we sometimes blame as bad timing, difficult times, or confusing circumstances may be the wise hand of God shaping our growth for a purposeful outcome.

This week we'll separate the three systems and put some fences around what we know. If disciplining, sifting, and pruning are part of God's plan to move us from marginal believers to powerful lovers of Christ, then together, we'll forge ahead to grasp this knowledge and let his systems do their work.

—— DAY 1: LEARNING TO LOVE THE "D" WORD

Lord, You have placed me where I am right now to influence others for Your kingdom by living out my faith. Thank You for creating and trusting me for this privilege. Amen.

Some words ambush us and hold a predictable response of dread. Discipline is one of these words. Many teachers try to console us by pointing out the word "disciple" is neatly tucked inside this word—but knowing that doesn't sway the dread I feel. I want to be a good disciple of the Lord more than I want to breathe, but for some reason I can't make the connection. In my mind discipline seems hard and often is yoked to punishment. I don't know anyone who rallies around hard, punishing things and calls them nice. The problem is we don't fully understand God's first system of growth—discipline.

No study of this word can begin without first understanding scripture. Please turn to our memory verse for the week—Hebrews 12:11 and then read verses 12-13 as well.

How is discipline described? What does it produce in those who allow it to work in their lives?

It's important to realize the only time discipline is necessary is when someone or something is about to take a turn that could impede growth. To our Father discipline equals protection. This is worth stopping and resting for a minute. Fill in the blank below.

DISCIPLINE = _____

For some reason we view discipline as harsh punishment, but truly, God only disciplines us to protect us from anything that might lure us away from him. Let's think about some of God's protective discipline in a realistic way.

Brittany has a habit of spreading negative words about people, even close friends, and one day she gets caught in the gossip. A close friend is hurt because of her actions and it causes distance between them. God disciplines Brittany by revealing her habit and gives her a chance to make things right with her friend, as well as make better choices in her conversations. This protects her reputation as a friend and bolsters her ability to lead and love other women.

Mark cheats in his business transactions, not reporting certain things to the IRS and withholding the truth from his accountants. He rationalizes that everyone else does it, and why should he give more of his money away to a government that doesn't deserve it? God allows Mark's accountants and peers to question him on some of his policies. They speak the truth to him and encourage him to make things right. This is God's way of protecting Mark from serious penalties if left unchanged.

Cathy continues to overeat and make poor choices with food. Her weight has steadily climbed over the years, and every now and then she drops ten pounds but quickly gains it back—adding to her frustration. Her doctor tells her she needs to lose weight to maintain good health, and her husband is frightened by her disregard for the warnings. God gives Cathy chances to change. He disciplines her by allowing her body to scream the warning signs that are visible to everyone around her. God is protecting her from the hardship of living in a body that carries too much weight, but it's up to her to pay attention to the protection. If she ignores it, she makes the choice to do things her way with imminent danger to her body and health.

In these scenarios it's how they respond to the discipline (protection) that matters, not the fact they've gotten themselves into these situations and don't know how to get out. God always provides a way out or a path of change, while the enemy keeps us paralyzed or blinded right where we are. Typically, we respond to discipline in one of four ways: we accept it with bitterness, we accept it with self-pity—thinking we don't really deserve it—we're angry and resent God for it, or we accept it gratefully as the appropriate response to a loving Father.[1]

Reflect for a moment on your own life. How do you receive discipline? Why do you think you react this way?

Now please turn to Revelation 3:19-20. Please write verse 19 below.

One Bible translation says it like this: "I continually discipline...so you can turn from your indifference and become enthusiastic about the things of God."[1] Oh—the difference between indifference and enthusiasm is paramount. In this passage Jesus warned the church in Laodicea that a lukewarm attitude towards the things that matter to God provokes Jesus to want to spit! We need to remember that God's purpose in discipline is protection. He doesn't want to harshly punish, but to bring us back into his loving care.

This scripture from Matthew is rich with meaning when it comes to discipline. It's also one of the hardest scriptures to truly understand.

> "So if your eye—even if it is your best eye!—causes you to lust, gouge it out and throw it away. ... And if your hand—even your right hand—causes you to sin, cut it off and throw it away. Better that than find yourself in hell." (Matthew 5:29-30 TLB)

How's that for bedtime reading? The words sound harsh yet they're essential if we're to grow. Was Matthew telling us Jesus said to poke out our eyes and cut off our hands? No, but he was trying to make a strong point. He was explaining that when God disciplines us for protection and we continue to wink at sin, the sins will eventually harm us. Let's recall our definition of sin in an earlier chapter: deliberate and emphatic independence of God. So, Jesus was figuratively saying if your eye (what you see, watch, believe) or hand (what you reach for, hold on to, grasp tightly) is causing you to move independently away from God, it's better to live with only one eye or hand than to remain unchanged and outside of his protective care.

Here's the beauty of the whole thing. The minute we ask God for protection or let go of our controlling grasp, He rides the heavens to our rescue.

Turn to Psalm 145:14-16. How does this scripture encourage you?

_____

_____

Oswald Chambers says, "God's Spirit alters the atmosphere of our way of looking at things, and things begin to be possible which never were possible before. Getting into the stride of God means nothing less than union with Himself. It takes a long time to get there—but keep at it. Don't give in because the pain is bad just now, get on with it, and before long you will find you have a new vision and a new purpose."

Father, I realize that to you, discipline is protection. You're a good Father who thinks only of my maturity and growth. Forgive me for the times I push your protection away. Thank You for loving me so wisely. Amen.

—— DAY 2: BECOMING GOOD TEST TAKERS

Lord Jesus, let Your loving discipline fall on the willing soil of my heart. I want to live out my love for You with confidence and peace. Amen.

Yesterday we introduced the concept of God's three-way growth system—disciplining, sifting, and pruning. As we focus again today on the ways of discipline, it's refreshing to note that discipline is an act of love that takes place within a family. Often, we confuse discipline with punishment. In her beautiful book Secrets of The Vine for Women, Darlene Wilkinson says, "Discipline is for God's children; punishment is for his enemies. Punishment includes anger, wrath, and the intent to make someone pay for their offenses. When Christ hung on the cross over two thousand years ago, he took on the punishment we all deserve for sin. The moment we believe by faith that through his death and resurrection Jesus paid the full penalty for our sins, the word punishment ceases to apply to us."[2]

What a relief it is to know we don't have to continually pay for everything we do that's wrong. If you're reading this and have never heard this good news, take off your shoes and dance. For those new to the idea of a personal love and relationship with Jesus Christ, you simply need to ask him to be Lord and to wash away the old for the new. That's it. The Bible says "...confess with your mouth Jesus as Lord, and believe in your heart that God raised him from the dead, and you will be saved. ...Whoever believes in Him will not be disappointed" (Romans 10:9,11 NASB).

When we're in the family of God, discipline becomes a gift rather than something we fear. Good parents discipline in ways that mold excellent children. How much more will God do in us who believe?

So, as we grow in the ways of discipline, God will provide checkpoints or markers along the way. These checkpoints give us a chance to show that what He has been teaching us has taken root. The Bible calls these checkpoints tests. For those of us who were never good test takers, don't worry. When God bring us to a checkpoint, he has given us every resource and training to be successful. As we mature, the tests we encounter actually give us a chance to show off for God.

Turn to James 1:2-4. What does the testing of our faith produce?

Look at 2 Corinthians 13:5-8. In this passage Paul exhorted the church in Corinth because its people were going through challenges of misguided behavior within the body, even to the point of mistrusting Paul's words to them. He challenged them to do something in verse 5. What was it?

Paul reminded the church that Jesus is in them. We, too, must allow the testing of our faith to produce mature results. It's helpful to note that pliable people are better test takers. When we're pliable, we're teachable—less defensive and proud. The church in Corinth was justifying all kinds of poor behavior and attitudes. Paul kept disciplining them with love (1 Corinthians 13).

Are you pliable when it comes to God's discipline? If not, why?

Now turn to 1 Peter 1:6-8. What happens when our faith is tested (vs. 7)?

This kind of test isn't exclusive to our salvation but extends to every chance we're given to overcome what has formally overcome us. As God reveals things that need to change or be put to death, we get to grow in our faith by passing the tests. Tests are the moments we make a choice. I'll either overeat—or walk away and praise. *I'll either gossip—or speak words of life. I'll either lash out and be offended—or extend grace to the offender.*

There's nothing like getting an A on a test. But even if we get a C (or an F if we totally blow it)—God is a God of retakes.

The book of Genesis holds one of the greatest tests of all time. Abraham, a man of great faith but costly mistakes, was brought to a point of maturity, faith, and surrender. He passed the test, and the discipline and shaping of God had its reward, but oh... how this story resonates.

Turn to Genesis 22:1-2. What has God brought Abraham to in his faith?

In order to understand the breadth of this test, we must understand what it meant to Abraham. Turn back to Genesis 15:1-6. What was God's promise to Abraham and how was this promise confusing to him?

At the time Abram (not yet changed to Abraham) believed God, even though he couldn't see the physical outcome of the promise in his present circumstances. I love how God was pleased with this faith and credited it him as "right living." But...the plague of time plundered his faith as it often does ours. When things don't happen quickly or within the timeframes we've prayed and hoped for, either our faith weakens or we try to help God along with the timing.

Turn to Genesis 16:1-4. How did both Abram and Sarai take matters into their own hands? Because we're focusing on Abram, what was his role in this decision?

Horrible, horrible mistakes all around! Sarai got impatient and panicked, and Abram foolishly said, "Sure, I'll sleep with your maid." As the story progressed, Hagar, Sarai's maid did get pregnant and gave birth. However, things we try to manipulate and pretend are faith rarely turn out how we expect. Eventually Sarah and Abraham had their own son as the Lord promised, and they named him Isaac. Things were wonderful until one day, the God Abraham loved asked the toughest question Abraham would ever face: "Are you willing to sacrifice your only true son?"

Please read all of Genesis 22 and pay attention to the holy tension of Abraham's faith and God's protective love. When did Abraham leave after hearing from God (vs. 3)?

Notice he did not form a committee to pray about this or journal for months. He heard and he moved. Sometimes we need to actively pray and wait, but other times we need to move. Only the Spirit can show us the difference. I believe the reason he was able to move so quickly in obedience to this test was he was trained (from passing so many other tests) to trust the goodness of God. He knew there would somehow be good resolution.

What did Abraham note in verse 8 when responding to his son?

This is important. When God brings a test, we're prepared and equipped for a good outcome. Abraham had endured many other tests and failed (lying about the status of his wife as they traveled, not once, but twice—sleeping with his wife's maid instead of leading his family well). Yet, when faced with being asked to give up the greatest joy and security of his life, he willingly obeyed. He'd been down the path of discipline before and knew its positive rewards. Whatever God was doing in him and through him, he trusted the process.

Please know that child sacrifice was an abomination to the Lord (Leviticus 18:21). God took no pleasure in seeing a boy strapped to an altar. Centuries later God the Father Himself would go through with this exact scene as his own son was brutally tortured and slain. This scene is often called a foreshadowing of Christ, and I believe in heaven Abraham will say it was his greatest honor to be tested in this way and pass. However, I can't imagine anything harder in the moment.

Let's think for a second about that phrase in the moment. When we're facing a test, it's that moment that counts. The moment the donuts are laid before you. The moment you stare down a menu and select. The moment you walk into an exercise class or ignore the prod to move. The moment you can bless with your words or curse. The moment you choose purity over compromise. Tests are built on those moments. Do you recognize your moments? What do you do in the heat of them?

How we handle our moments determines the outcome of our tests. What was the outcome of Abraham's moment in verses 15-18?

Friends, our tests will look different from Abraham's, but the aftermath is the same. Our moments of testing hold the key to our future and our faith. May we test well. *My Father, I understand that discipline and testing come to mature me not to harm me or mock my faith. I pray for power and boldness to face my moments of testing and to make You proud. Amen.*

—— DAY 3: SIFTED BUT NOT OVERCOME
Jesus, I give you this day to learn new concepts and fresh ways of understanding Your truth. Give me spiritual eyes to see and to hear. Amen.

This week we're focused on the growth strategies our Father uses to bring us to maturity—disciplining, sifting, and pruning. We spent Day One and Day Two on the concept of discipline and tests. Today we'll look at the concept of **sifting**.

Throughout the Bible the word sift is used to describe the process of wheat being taken from stalks to become the useful grain used to nourish. In biblical times the stalk was cut down by the reapers, gleaned, and placed into bundles—then thrown on a threshing floor to be crushed. As the wheat was crushed, the good part of the stalk was separated from the bad and the useful parts were gathered to be distributed for sustenance. The difficult latter part of this process is called sifting.

In heaven's vocabulary sifting has a God-ordained purpose, but it originates with Satan himself. The Bible shares two poignant examples of sifting that we'll study today.

Please turn to Luke 22:31-34. What did Jesus tell Peter in verse 31?

The beautiful scene of the Last Supper ended with an unexpected turn for Peter. Jesus informed him Satan had asked (the NASB version uses demanded) to sift him like wheat. What does this mean? Earlier in our chapters we looked at Revelation 12:10 where Satan is called the accuser, standing before the throne of God day and night accusing the brethren. We also studied the schemes of the devil. Because he is not all-powerful or all-knowing, he can only study our action and reaction to things in order to build a strategy against us. I've studied Peter more than anyone in the New Testament, perhaps because I'm a lot like him. He tended to struggle with the approval of men and also enjoyed the drama and heroics of Jesus. When they were feeding multitudes, he was thrilled, but when Jesus spoke of the cross he said, "Let it never be!" Satan went right for Peter's jugular—trying to take him out of the game completely—but Jesus had the final say.

What did Jesus tell Peter he did after Satan asked to sift him (vs. 32)?

Before we continue with how that night ended for Peter, we need to press into the fact that Satan demanded to sift Peter, and in God's infinite wisdom...He said "yes." At first glance we may be tempted to question God on that one. Isn't he loving? Doesn't he protect us from evil? Yes, and yes. But there are times when he allows the enemy to sift us, so we'll mature at an accelerated rate.

Remember Job and the hedge of protection we studied in Week 7? There's another example of Satan asking God to put a believer through a time of sifting—and God answered "yes." In Job's case it meant losing much of what he valued and put his life efforts towards. In Peter the sifting was a personal assault on his character.
When it comes to growth strategies, discipling and pruning are done by the gentle hands of God. Sifting is done by the harsh and demeaning wiles of Satan.

Turn to Matthew 26:69-75. How did this sifting take place later the same night?

Peter was one of Jesus's best friends. Satan knew Peter struggled with approval, and in that instant, the approval of servants was more important than the approval of his Lord.

Let's try to make this concept of sifting personal. I'm emerging from one of the most painful sifting periods of my life. I've mentioned the difficult time I've had in Uganda with our precious ministry The Vine. In the past months I had to let go three of our top employees, including my co-founder, who was like a son to me. Betrayal, lies, deceit... all part of the package. In the midst of this trying time, I was sifted and crushed as the enemy relentlessly reminded me of my own mistakes. I hashed and rehashed them—and at times felt like quitting, even though many of the world's most vulnerable women and children would languish without our care. I endured taunts, death threats, a bizarre foreign legal system, and mental anguish too intense to describe.

Why would God allow such sifting when the goal was only to help others and bring the good news to the ends of the earth? Growth—plain and simple. I'm not the same woman, leader, or lover of Christ that I was six months ago. Truthfully, I'll never be the same.

When Satan sifts us for destruction, we must trust our Lord to bring re-construction. People often ask, "How do I know if it's sifting, disciplining, or pruning?" Believe me, sifting has a cruel and harsh edge to it, while disciplining and pruning have a loving and purposeful tone.

Think about your own life. Are you in a season of sifting? Is there a harsh or demanding set of circumstances taking a toll on you? If not now, can you think of a time there was?

The key to a time of sifting is to draw to the heart of the Father like never before. Sit quietly before him and whisper praise for his goodness. Lean into trusting and abandoned prayer rather than forceful demands for blessing and outcomes. Remember, Job lost everything including his health and yet trusted the goodness of God.

For Peter the days of Jesus's crucifixion were probably a blur of remorse and harsh sifting. Notice we don't see him at the cross or by Mary's side. Where was he? Probably crying and lamenting in an upper room. But then we see a brilliant scene of restoration.

Please read John 21: 1-17. How did Jesus surprise and restore Peter in this chapter?

The good news about sifting is God never allows us to remain crushed wheat on the floor. He gently scoops us up and wipes off the dirt, then gives us a brilliant purpose— becoming nourishment for others.

Father, You are so beautiful and loving. Your purpose and kind will overshadow any scheme of the enemy. Amen.

—— DAY 4: WHY WE NEED TO BE PRUNED

Jesus, Your words to the disciples are life. You are the vine and we are the branches. Without You, we can do nothing. Amen.

So far, we've studied the concept of God's growth strategy in our lives—disciplining and sifting. The rest of this week we'll focus on the necessary act of pruning.

Pruning is a gardening term, and for the life of me, I'm not a gardener. I've planted rose bushes and can mow a lawn with the best of them...but when it comes to really understanding the growth of plants, I'm lost. I'll never forget when Bobby took the rose bushes I'd planted and pruned them back to mere branches. I almost fainted! They looked good to me as they were. They even had a few pretty roses blooming at the time. Bobby learned from his father, who kept a meticulous garden, that if you don't prune back the leaves and even the blossoms of a bush at given times—the blossoms and fruit to come will be small and straggly. Pruning enables the greatest nutritional flow to reach all parts of the branch so it's ready and able to produce the best fruit, not just some fruit. In my ignorance, I would have settled for some.

Let's start by reading Jesus's words about pruning. Even if you've read these verses many times, the Spirit wants us to continue to learn from them in a deeper way. Pray to see and hear with a fresh desire for growth.

Please read John 15:1-5. Let's determine who's who in these verses. Please note who is the vinedresser, who is the vine, and who are the branches.

This conversation took place immediately following the Last Supper. If you glance at John 14:31, you see that Jesus said, "Let's go...." We know they walked through the lush vineyards of the Kidron Valley on their way to the Garden of Gethsemane, and Jesus used this scenery for some of the most stunning

teaching we have on growth in the entire Bible. Remember, Jesus was talking to believers here. He was speaking to those who understood that knowing and loving

Him impacts the world. But He was also aware of the confusion His words brought. I can imagine the twisted faces of the disciples as He talked about branches being cut off and pruned to bear more fruit. He quickly had to assure them they were all clean and ready for useful service (verse 3), because immediately they probably felt as we do at times: "I'm not worthy...I'm not good enough...you need to pick someone else." The picture of cutting away so more can come is a brilliant strategy God has chosen to bring growth and influence from those who love Him.

To be clear, pruning is different from disciplining, although both come from the hand of God. Darlene Wilkinson clearly separates the two in the following way:[2]

» Disciplining brings pain (you're acting in such a way that God must intervene to stop sin or waywardness for your protection) while pruning brings discomfort (necessary for new growth).
» The Vinedresser (God) has one intent: whereas in discipline he longs to bring fruit, in pruning he longs for us to bear more fruit.
» When we are disciplined sin must go (disobeying God), but when we are pruned self must go (putting ourselves before God).
» Our rightful response to discipline should be repentance (turn away from sin), while our best response to pruning is release (surrender to God).[3]

Knowing the difference between these two helps us understand the growth strategy of our father. During a season of pruning, it helps to know that God is taking us to a new place of abundance we've not been able to get to prior to this season. His goal is abundance while ours is often relief.

Turn to John 10:10. What is Jesus' ultimate purpose in our lives?

Read Ephesians 3:20. What's happening as we grow?

We can't even think to ask all that God wants to do for us and in us. Our minds aren't even big enough to grasp it. Pruning goes hand in hand with God's glory being show-cased in our lives and his kingdom advancing through our humility and strength. As we welcome pruning rather than fight it, we begin to experience the purpose of our lives: to grow in our love and enjoyment of God. His love for us never changes based on our behavior or submission to the pruning shears—but our love for Him deepens as we trust the Vinedresser to take away whatever He must so we may thrive.

In a tender letter from Paul to a young man he loved in the faith named Titus, he masterfully painted the notion of godly living from a scaffold we can understand.

Turn to Titus 3:1-8. List as many things as you can from these verses that indicate mature living.

Paul ended these verses by saying, "I want to stress these things, so that those who have trusted in God may be careful to devote themselves to doing what is good. These things are excellent and profitable for everyone" (Titus 3:8 NIV).

Knowing that God's goal is what's excellent and profitable for everyone, let's make pruning a bit more personal. Typically, God prunes us in one of the following ways:

- Priorities that need to be rearranged
- Relationships that need to change or end
- Busyness that isn't accomplishing what matters most
- Dependencies or attachments that we're ready to grow out of
- Personal "rights" that God is asking us to surrender to Him

Let's take a moment to quietly ask God what he may be pruning in our lives. Are there any areas we need to sway towards his loving shears for more growth?

As we close our time today, I want to encourage you to not be afraid of pruning. It's the excellent way of the vinedresser—and leads us to a harvest beyond compare.

Father, You are loving and wise. Everything about You is good. If You take something from us, it's always to be replaced with an abundance of harvest growth. Amen.

—— DAY 5: A LIFE OF ABUNDANCE

Father, as a loving vinedresser, I long to bear more fruit, but confess I'm not sure how. With anticipation, I learn from your perfect ways. Amen.

Jesus gave an interesting example when he mentioned the cure for anxiety in the Gospel of Matthew. He said, "Observe how the lilies of the field grow; they do not toil nor do they spin..." (Matthew 6:28, NASB). Can you imagine a lily straining within itself to grow? "Oh, I must reach a certain height! Every other lily around me seems to be doing great! I hate my leaves and my stem and my blossom...why can't my petals look more like the flower next to me?" Sounds ridiculous to think of a lily lamenting about how it grows, yet Jesus gave this example to show us this mentality is ridiculous.

The joy of producing much fruit after a season of pruning is promised. Pruning means we allow God to remove or reshape something now to become more beautiful later. There are only two things we must do in the process of pruning: allow our vine-dresser full access with his loving shears and stay closely connected to the vine—our precious Jesus.

Let's go back to our anchor scripture for this teaching in the gospel of John. Please read John 15:7-8. What is the requirement described for bearing much fruit?

Some translations use the word remain, but a better rendering of the word used there is abide. To abide means to live in, breathe in, exist in, be comfortable within. Virtually, Jesus promises if we live and breathe in Him, if His words of hope and promise exist within us, if we're so comfortable with Him that anything else pales in comparison, we can ask whatever we wish, and it will be done. The results of abiding are we will bear much fruit and prove that we're truly disciples of our Lord.

Most of us have heard this description before but wonder: "What does it look like to abide?"

Turn to the following scriptures and note what God promises to those who long to abide in Him.

Psalm 57:1-3:

Joshua 1:5-9,13:

_____

_____

1 John 3:1-3:

_____

_____

According to scripture, as we abide we need only to realize that God will accomplish what concerns us as we courageously trust Him. We are His, and nothing can diminish or harm our abiding. It is a holy place of trust.

If abiding is the prerequisite for bearing much fruit, let's look at the practical steps we take to abide.

We set our time and love for Jesus apart from serving him.
One of Jesus's great friends, Martha, learned this in a blunt way. Turn to Luke 10:38. Who invited Jesus to have dinner that night and welcomed him into her home?

_____

_____

Scripture notes it was Martha. She was the friendly mover and shaker of Bethany. The one who made it happen from appetizer to dessert to candles on the table. Yet, look what Jesus said to her in verses 41-42. He was sitting right there and she was serving him like crazy, but there is no abiding happening whatsoever—only the frenzied pace of getting things done. It's like hosting a party for someone and forgetting they're there. Hard to imagine, but I do it all the time.

Honestly reflect on your abiding time. This is the time you sit quiet, pushing aside all noise and the pace of frenzy. Perhaps you have the Bible open and learn from certain scriptures as you abide—not to check in the box of a study accomplished or a group you need to prepare for—but rather, as the greatest book of secrets ever written. Secrets that unfold in this time of abiding and bloom into knowledge, wisdom, and discernment you didn't possess before.

In Luke 10:42 Jesus explained to Martha there is something precious about this abiding time she was missing. How did he describe the difference between Martha's pursuits and Mary's?

When we spend time abiding rather than performing, rushing, or demanding things line up in our dictated manner, a great joy overtakes us as we experience the pleasure of being in the company of God.

Abiding in Jesus is intentional, and with practice, becomes natural.
To truly be one who abides, we welcome pruning as the catalyst to a greater sense of relationship.

Abiding with Jesus doesn't magically happen. Our feeble brains are too scattered for that to be true. Think about how many times our mind wanders while we pray. Or how we become the point of what we wanted to offer to God. Don't worry: abiding isn't natural in the beginning—it's intentional. We intentionally push things out of our mind and say they can wait. We intentionally focus on the attributes and beauty of our King rather than the reality of the fallen world around us. We intentionally pray as a love language rather than a reward language. You get the point. The more we're intentional and think of abiding as a state of being rather than doing, we're on our way. Pruning helps us get there.

Turn to Joshua 5:1-9. After the miraculous venture of marching through the Jordan River toward the promised land—spirits were high and emotions elated. The Israelites were finally getting their forty-year promise. But suddenly, on the verge of this great fete, God demanded an unexpected offering. A pruning of large proportion.

What did the Lord ask Joshua to do, and what did He demand of the Israelites (vs. 2-5)?

What did the Lord say to Joshua in verse 9, and what was the name of the place of their circumcision?

Gilgal means "to end," and in a stunning act of "cutting away" (circumcision), his people were ready to finally enter what had long been promised. Several things had to happen for God's purpose to go forth. The cutting away was a sharp reminder that this promise was from God, not something they created themselves. This act of being set apart led to a quiet time of healing (vs. 8), when everyone had to remain in the camp until they were ready to move on. I imagine this time was reflective—a time they joined together as a community, as well as personally abided in praise and the awe of His presence. Pain has a way of pushing us there.

Note what happened after this time of abiding and pruning in verses 11-12.

As the Israelites let the work of pruning settle them into a deeper (or perhaps for some a new) way of abiding, lives were ready for the old way of sustenance to cease and a new way to be provided. They simply couldn't get there any other way, and neither can we. Abiding is the ultimate mark of maturity. It's the sweet scent of a life that's been disciplined and pruned for more growth.

Use these tips to help with abiding:
- Set aside time throughout the day not for regimented study or prayer, but rather, for listening and quiet inner praise. (Of course, still study and pray. I'm merely saying that abiding is not something we do for God, but rather for the practice of enjoying and listening. Certainly, this happens when we study and pray, but those times can become ruts of obedience. I'm proposing abiding to be a fresh time of awareness and love.)
- The minute something arises that causes stress or fear, shut your eyes (unless you're driving) and quietly vow to trust rather than worry—to believe rather than fret and spiral into despair.
- Offer a time of mindless activity to the Lord for abiding prayer. It might be

washing the dishes, doing chores, a time you'd normally watch a TV show you don't really care about, a drive from one place to the next. Whatever you like... use it as an inner sanctuary for personal communion with Go

- Don't be afraid of pruning. Instead, welcome it. Tell the Lord often that He may have His way with you...knowing it will yield a stronger life, filled with more fruit than you can imagine.

Lord, have Your way in me. You may set me apart for Your purposes as I desire nothing but to abide in You. Amen.

—— DAY 6: REFLECTION AND APPLICATION

Jesus, You are the power, purpose, and point of my life. I'm excited to see the growth You bring as I lay down my life for Yours. Amen.

This week we talked about the growth strategy of our Lord and how He uses disciplining, sifting, and pruning to bring us to maturity. In a journal, write the words disciplining, sifting, and pruning as the heading of three columns. In each column fill in time periods when you know God allowed or worked within the events of your life for a fruitful outcome. If you're currently in the midst of one of these time periods, write a prayer to the Lord allowing Him to do whatever it takes to get you to a point of abiding in Him and bearing much fruit for his purposes. Share this prayer with your prayer partner so she can pray it alongside you.

Holy Spirit, I trust You are working for my growth in ways I don't recognize. Open my eyes to see that what looks like pain is often the grasp of Your purposeful teaching. Amen.

—— DAY 7: REFLECTION AND APPLICATION

Father, this week has been a beautiful reminder of who You are and the desire You have that longs for me to grow. May I want to grow as much as You want to help me get there. Amen.

This week we singled out John 15 as we studied the idea of pruning and abiding, but it's fascinat-ing to read the entire content of Jesus's last night with his disciples as one reading. Today, go back to the Gospel of John and read chapters 13-17 if you have the time. Read it without stopping, try-ing to imagine how it felt to hear all this teaching in one night.

It began with an upper room supper and ended in the Kidron Valley vineyards in the ravine before entering the famous Garden of Gethsemane. Picture the places you would have sat as you listened to Jesus talk. How would you have felt as he prayed the High Priestly Prayer in chapter 17? What mood would you have been in when the soldiers came to arrest Jesus?

In the margin of your Bible note the words that describe how you feel and the relevance of these verses to your life today. Put dates next to your words that will remind you of what the Holy Spirit is showing you as you absorb these chapters during this period of your life.

My Lord, I can only imagine what it would have been like to sit and learn at Your feet. How re-markable I can still learn in the same way by treasuring Your words in my Bible. Amen.

Notes

1. Life Application Bible (Wheaton, Ill.: Tyndale, 1988), commentary, 1912.

2. Adapted from Darlene Wilkinson, Secrets of the Vine for Women (New York: Multnomah Books, 2011), 58.

WEEK TEN: LIVING BEYOND FREE

SCRIPTURE MEMORY VERSE
May he give you the desire of your heart and make all your plans succeed.
Psalm 20:4

People often ask me what it's like to be free from food compulsion. One woman wondered, "Do you think about food all day and plan how you're not going to eat it?" I smiled at her gently and took my time with an answer. I wanted to make sure to convey what was in my heart—knowing her question revealed a lot about the hurt in hers. "Actually, I spend very little time thinking about food," I replied. "I enjoy it—and look forward to it when I'm hungry—but that's as far as it goes. My mind is engaged in so many more interesting things I don't really give it much thought." Her face twisted in a look of confusion as she sighed, "I can't imagine not thinking about food day and night. Your mind must feel so free."

Indeed, it does. But freedom is not to be hoarded. I've spent a good part of my adult life assuring people they, too, can be free. The problem is we talk about the wrong things. We dwell on willpower, self-control, and strategies to help us white-knuckle bear down and overcome a show-down with a strawberry glazed donut, while the root problem and solution stare us in the face. Turning from the dregs of gluttony to the free fields of grace is what we want to do. There's a whole world outside compulsion with food—and when you bravely decide to live there—you'll be living *Beyond Free*.

In my first book, *Be Free*, I laid the groundwork for freedom. If you haven't done that study, I encourage you to go back and complete it. It will help a lot of what we covered in this book make sense. This book was designed to take you deeper and move you farther out on the horizon of free-living. The concepts we covered are not for the faint of heart. But I've had the joy of cheering you on to glory...and now my voice is hoarse from yelling, "You can do it!"

So, as we come to our last week of study (there's still one more week of celebration), I want to keep things simple. Each day this week I'll take one word and we'll focus on it deeply. My hope is that by the end of Week Twelve, we'll not only understand we can *Be Free*, but we'll boldly desire to abide Beyond Free—for the rest of our lives.

—— DAY 1: HUNGER

Lord, help me to understand that I will never go hungry when I turn to You, because you are the bread of life. Amen.

True hunger is a bit confusing. In Africa it's the rhythm of life. I've held the worn hands of women who dig in potato fields trying to forage enough to feed their families. In America hunger is illusive and hard to define. We know it by the empty rumblings within, but easy access to food and a plethora of choices makes hunger something we're annoyed by, not something we learn from. For a good part of my life I ignored hunger. Like so many, I'd carry snacks and fill my days with mindless eating, never even considering hunger as an indicator as to when to eat, or heaven forbid, what or how much. To make matters worse, I never realized there's a physical hunger and a spirit hunger[1] to be considered. When our spirit is hungry and we feed our body instead, chaos begins.

Author Geneen Roth shares her lament,

> "When I first decided I wasn't going to diet anymore, I began keeping a chart of when I ate, what I ate, and if I was hungry. After a few days I was dismayed to realize that I never ate because I was hungry. There were too many other good reasons to eat: when I was upset and needed a treat; when I was happy and needed to celebrate; when I was sad and needed to be comforted; when I was angry and didn't express it; when I was in love and wanted to share. And, if none of the above applied, when I was frustrated or bored and couldn't figure out what else to do. Food was the glue that held my life together between hungers."[2]

How about you? Why do you eat?

In his farewell ceremonial address Moses spoke to the Israelites in a way that would stir and comfort them. Let's look at what God has to say about true hunger.

Read Deuteronomy 8:1-3. What were some of the purposes mentioned in these verses for their years of wandering (vs. 1-2)?

Please write verse 3 below and circle the phrase with the word hunger in it.

What was said to God's people then is still true for us today. He humbles us and allows us to become hungry, so we can be fed by *His manna*—a manna that is more than bread or tasty delight but comes from His mouth and satisfies every inner rumble or desire of our soul.

Read Matthew 4:4. How was this scripture used by Jesus when he was hungry?

Now let's turn to John 6:1-58. Watch the role of hunger and feeding play out through the eyes of Jesus. How did Jesus react to man's need to be filled (vs. 1-14)?

How did the people react to being fed (vs. 14)?

In verses 15-25 the crowd that followed Jesus to the other side of the sea were the ones who were fed and filled the day before. Notice it doesn't say the healed followed him but those who came back to the place they were fed.

This is a strong reminder that our hunger for God goes much deeper than our stomachs. It even outweighs the dramatic miracles we long for from God—reminding us of the simplicity of the cadence of being hungry, then filled. Hungry...then filled. Hungry...then filled.

If we pay attention, we'll keep coming back to the shore of our deepening relationship—a longing to hear more, learn more, be touched—again and again.

Next, we experience what may be the most powerful teaching on food in the Bible in John 6:26-35. What did he say to the crowd in verse 27?

To help his Jewish brothers and sisters better understand, he gave some background about manna—but then he redefined the whole notion of food.
What did he proclaim in verse 35?

In the previous verses Jesus explained there are two types of food: food that is perishing (what we eat daily, what we plan for and obsess over) and food that endures to eternal life. If we spend most of our lives trying to tame the first kind of food, we may be malnourished when it comes to the second, Jesus, the Bread of Life.

If I'm honest, I know there are times I'm feeding myself with no regard to my spirit hunger or the calm assurance that Jesus is the true bread of life, not Panera. But in my freedom, there's a sweet sanity that knows the difference—and consistently makes the right choice to observe and reflect before stuffing my face with food that's not necessary.

How do you see yourself? Are you aware of hunger or masking it with continual, mindless eating?

This is a strong reminder that our hunger for God goes much deeper than our stomachs. It even outweighs the dramatic miracles we long for from God—reminding us of the simplicity of the cadence of being hungry, then filled. Hungry...then filled. Hungry...then filled.

If we pay attention, we'll keep coming back to the shore of our deepening relationship—a longing to hear more, learn more, be touched—again and again.

Next, we experience what may be the most powerful teaching on food in the Bible in John 6:26-35. What did he say to the crowd in verse 27?

To help his Jewish brothers and sisters better understand, he gave some background about manna—but then he redefined the whole notion of food. What did he proclaim in verse 35?

In the previous verses Jesus explained there are two types of food: food that is perishing (what we eat daily, what we plan for and obsess over) and food that endures to eternal life. If we spend most of our lives trying to tame the first kind of food, we may be malnourished when it comes to the second, Jesus, the Bread of Life.

If I'm honest, I know there are times I'm feeding myself with no regard to my spirit hunger or the calm assurance that Jesus is the true bread of life, not Panera. But in my freedom, there's a sweet sanity that knows the difference—and consistently makes the right choice to observe and reflect before stuffing my face with food that's not necessary.

How do you see yourself? Are you aware of hunger or masking it with continual, mindless eating?

If Jesus were dining with you, explaining He is the Bread of Life, do you think you'd really want to overeat the crumbs and morsels that are second best?

_____

_____

_____

Jesus, I know you're the Bread of Life, but I long to understand what that really means. Replace my desire for excessive food with a lavish desire to feast on You. Amen.

—— DAY 2: TABLE

I've often thought that in any home the table may be the most important piece of furniture. The table is where we gather. We sit and talk, share, dream, cry. We break bread and study at a table. We sip coffee and let our minds wander. We catch up on events and hold hands to pray. The table has a heartbeat. Its pulse is alive with purpose as it beckons us to sit down and dine richly in solitude or in good company.

It's no accident the Lord used a table to speak to his disciples the last night he spent with them before the cross, and a table is the imagery God used as something he prepares for us who trust him and wait. To live Beyond Free we must start to view the table as something more than a place to eat.

Please turn to Hebrews 9:1-4. Where was the consecrated bread located and what was that place called (vs. 2)?

_____

_____

_____

Where was the manna in a jar located and what was that place in the tent called (vs. 4)?

_____

_____

_____

This portion of scripture is often labeled "The Old and the New." I used to skip chunks of scripture like this thinking they weren't relevant now that Jesus has come—but the table in this scripture is relevant. Notice what sat on the table: the consecrated bread. Then, tucked into the presence of God in the Ark of the Covenant was a jar of the manna God provided in the wilderness. Bread on a table and manna in a jar—both are signs that God provides, which is absolutely enough.

According to Jewish history, the table's purpose was to hold the twelve loaves of bread called shewbread. The literal meaning of this word is "bread set out before the face and presence of God." Before Jesus became the Bread of Life, there was bread symbolizing the very face of God towards us, His people.

Continue to read Hebrews 9:8-14. What is the Holy Spirit trying to convey in verses 8-10?

_____

_____

_____

No matter how many times the priests put shewbread on the table and made sacrifice for sin—it was never enough—not until Jesus and his blood on the cross cleansed our conscience once and for all (vs. 14). Now the Bread of Life invites us to a different type of table.

Turn to Luke 22:14 then 24-30. How did Jesus define the greatest and least who sat around His table?

_____

_____

_____

In Hebrews we looked at the role of the old bread placed at the table; in Luke we looked at the role of the bread at the new table. Jesus explained that some of the things we think are great need to be redefined. Can you imagine on the very same night Jesus washed the disciples' feet, they entered a heated discussion on who was the greatest in God's kingdom? However, a desire for attention was not all he was exposing at that table. Ultimately, he exposed anything that shoves itself in the way of honest humility.

Let's take this one step further. Jesus asked the disciples, "Who is greater, the waiter or the one he serves?" Of course, we'd all say the one who orders from the menu and is served. But Jesus said he made himself the waiter, serving us—and it's a higher position than eating and drinking at the table.

I wonder how many of us might miss this encounter because we're too busy fretting over the meal more than the server. We may not even notice the server and fixate on the burger or pasta we can't wait to ingest. How will the meal be prepared? What about dessert? Jesus invites us to something real and deep (becoming a servant, like Him), so we don't want to miss it with our heads buried in food.

Does food, weight, or a poor self-image keep you from serving Jesus in a higher capacity than you are today?

If weight or food compulsion were not in the picture, what are the things you'd like to do? Imagine serving Jesus with every desire within you. What would that look like?

The wonderful thing about God is He understands how hard all of this is. That's why He gives us promises and encouragement in his Word. For another look at a table today, let's turn to Psalm 23.

Please read the entire psalm and write verse 5 below.

I've meditated on this verse a thousand times in the past few months. What interests me most is God says He prepares a table for us in the presence of our enemies—not in a back room or a private setting but in the presence of everything that's hard. In the presence of voices that taunt. In the presence of past mistakes and future victories. In the presence of smells and sights and temptations. He sets a beautiful table with china, candles, cloth napkins, and a place card with a stunning rendering of your name in gold ink. Then, as if that weren't enough—He pulls up a chair and sits down at the table with you to dine.

What's your "In the presence of...?" What is making it hard for you to succeed (voices, lack of desire or motivation, battling temptation with willpower rather than prayer and surrender)?

Write a table prayer below, thanking God for being our Bread of Life, our servant, and the One who prepares a table for us in the presence of our enemy.

Lord, I sit at the table with You in awe and praise. Everything You've prepared for me is life-giving and sustaining. Amen.

—— DAY 3: ALL IN

Jesus, You gave everything for me, how can I give anything less? I'm fully and completely Yours. Amen.

Being married to a professional athlete and coach has taught me a lot about commitment. At the beginning of a new baseball season, we can see how well the team will do by how committed the players and staff are in their efforts to win. If the commitment level is small to marginal—the results will be too! If the commitment is strong, we're assured the team will excel. We call this commitment playing "All In."

As I've matured spiritually, I've noticed the same principles apply. If we jump in and fully emerge ourselves in the efforts to surrender, change, and grow—the results will be stunning. But, if we continue with one foot in and one foot out—always leaving room for excuses and self-sabotage—we won't experience the joy of All In. Nothing compares to knowing we've given all we have to emerge fully transformed.

There's a woman tucked away in a well-known scripture that went All In. As a matter of fact, she gave so lavishly to Jesus that the respected men and disciples made fun of her and rebuked her!

Please turn to Mark 14:1-11. What did this woman do in verse 3 that caused such a stir?

This scripture is mentioned in the other gospels, but scholars continue to study to clarify some of the details. Some believe that Simon the Leper was the father of Martha, Mary, and Lazarus. Everyone agrees that Simon couldn't possibly have still struggle with leprosy because lepers weren't allowed in the city gates, let alone able to have houseguests. Because this dinner took place in Bethany, the hometown of Jesus's closest friends, it certainly could be that Jesus healed Simon in the past, so now he was hosting a dinner in His honor. Whatever the case, the unnamed woman (we know it was Mary, the sister of Martha, due to John's reference in John 12) came with an alabaster vial of perfume. These alabaster vials were made of costly stone that resembles marble, but softer in texture. Most likely, she'd been collecting the beautiful perfume over time, as the total worth of what she offered was almost a year's worth of wages.

She waited for just the right moment, and there, in the presence of a large dinner party, broke the stone vial and began to pour the contents on Jesus's head. I can hear the embarrassed gasps as people watched perfume drip down the face of Jesus. What a nuisance! What a bother! Why is she messing up the vibe of a perfectly good gathering? But then Jesus spoke. What did Jesus explain in verses 6-9?

The heart of what Jesus taught that night is the heart of living All In for our Lord. Let's study this further.

She's done a good deed (vs. 6). After telling the shocked crowd to leave Mary alone, he complimented her by calling her actions good. Some translations use the word beautiful, which takes this comment to an even deeper place. So much of what we do for the Lord may seem like duty, drudgery, or a rote behavior we've done for so long in the same way—with no spark or real cost to the act. Jesus shut the mouths of the party by smiling with a dripping head and saying, "She's done a beautiful thing... let her be." Perhaps she was saving that vial for her wedding day or for an assurance of finances down the road—whatever the case, she poured it out on Jesus that very night, and she came to the party prepared to pour. She didn't bring the vial and hide it in her coat, waiting to see if the opportunity was right—she made the opportunity by stepping out towards the face of Jesus, and then she poured.

Make this personal. Is there a beautiful deed you need to pour onto the Lord today? Write it below. Don't wait. Do it swiftly.

She has done what she could (vs. 8). Ultimately, that's all God asks. Did we do what we could? Mary had no way of knowing what she did was prophetic and would be talked about for centuries to come. If she knew, it might have tainted her sacrifice. Jesus called her act a preparation for his burial. She was anointing the Son of God before he took on the sins of the world on the cross. But that night, all she did is what she could. She took what she had (perfume of great price) and gave it away to the one she loved. No fanfare, no drudgery, no white-knuckle confusion as she held tightly to the vial she valued. Lovingly and confidently Mary poured what she loved over the one she loved more than what she possessed—Jesus.

The memory of this woman will be the love she poured over Me (vs. 9). We rarely get to see the impact our love for Christ leaves on those around us, and you know what? I'm glad. Jesus spoke to something that lingers after our love. That night, as Jesus left the dinner party, the scent of Mary's love may have lasted until his arrest and death on the cross. Certainly, it remained on the clothes he wore, if not in his perfume drenched hair. Imagine: we leave a scent of Christ when we love him well, and he is anointed again and again as we pour out our affection daily on the one we love. This pouring isn't always the big things we do but often a myriad of smaller things.

What kind of scent are we leaving? Is it sweet and inviting—or strong and pungent?

As we close our time today, mediate on these verses from 2 Corinthians 2:14-16 (NASB).

"But thanks be to God, who always leads us in His triumph in Christ, and manifests through us the sweet aroma of the knowledge of Him in every place. For we are a fragrance of Christ to God among those who are being saved and among those who are perishing; to the one an aroma of death to death, to the other an aroma from life to life."

Lord, I long to pour out on You the sweetest aroma. Take all that I am as I pour my treasure onto You. Amen.

—— DAY 4: OLD AND NEW

Jesus, something in me longs to press towards what's new, and yet the old in me tugs too. Let the fresh new awakening I have toward you reign and the old tugs of the flesh simply melt away. Amen.

At the beginning of our study I mentioned that I've learned some of my greatest life lessons from food. There's not one embarrassing behavior with food that I haven't pitifully participated in. As I think back I realize food has taught me immeasurably about trust, self-control, and the search for something of far greater worth than momentary satisfaction. In other words, food has helped me to mature spiritually. It's not the food itself—because it's just food. But rather, it's been the intentional pursuit of God's heart and what it means to be truly filled. It's posturing myself to fall deeper in love with Jesus rather than the distraction of my taste buds and fleeting pleasure that soon backfires and brings shame. It's the offering of my life to be used for his purposes, rather than a food induced coma of lethargy and guilt.

In the book of Philippians, the apostle Paul takes us through these scriptures in the same manner. While food humbled me, I believe the thing that humbled Paul was his pride. He was truly on his way as a Pharisee, climbing the ranks of success and fame and doing whatever it took to get approval from those he respected. Then suddenly, on a dusty road to a city he was charging to for more destruction Jesus met him and blinded him so that he could truly see. From a jail cell, Paul wrote incredible words about the old and new.

Please turn to Philippians 3:7-11. In verse 8, what kind of things do you think Paul was referring to?

Basically, Paul was recollecting the things he used to think mattered and placing them against what he now knew was true. We've spent the past ten weeks evaluating what matters and what doesn't. As you reflect on your own life, what falls in the old category of importance and what lies in the new? I'll share some of my understanding to get us started.

OLD:

- I can eat what I want when I want because God is more concerned with my spirit than my body.
- I can separate my physical life and hunger from my spiritual life. The two don't really intersect.
- The way I posture myself to please God is to work harder, strive more. If I want to accomplish something I better get it done!

NEW:

- God cares about everything in my life, even the hairs on my head. My body is His home and I welcome Him in...body, soul, and spirit.
- Most of the hunger I experience is a hunger for God, not for food. As a matter of fact, I am easily satisfied when I feed my body's hunger—but the expanse of my spirit hunger is deep and always taking me deeper in love.
- The typical posture for weight loss is work harder, try more, stress and strain until results are seen. When the goal is freedom not merely weight loss, I'm invited to trust rather than more internal strain. I trust the Holy Spirit as He shows me truth—and my choices are seeds I sow for life rather than strain I feel towards failure.

Your turn:

OLD:

_____

_____

_____

_____

_____

NEW:

_____

_____

_____

_____

_____

Read verses 13-14. How did Paul give himself grace in this process rather than make excuses for failure?

_____

_____

Previously in verse 10, Paul referred four things: knowing Jesus intimately, understanding the power of life overcoming death, considering the hard times in life as fellowshipping with Jesus as we grasp the concept of suffering, and embracing the truth that as we die (our flesh, worldly views) a new and vibrant person emerges. He said he did not claim to be perfect at all this yet, but that he would keep pressing on (Philippians 4:12). Why? The reason is the most significant lesson we'll learn in our time on earth. Look back to verse 12 and reflect on this statement:

"To take hold of that for which Christ Jesus took hold of me."

Why did Jesus take hold of you? Have you stopped to think there are specific reasons for your life—with the ultimate reason being the pure and absolute enjoyment of loving and knowing God as your Father, Jesus as your Savior, and the Holy Spirit as the friend who teaches and leads in the sweetest of ways? Some of you will teach others how to be free from the freedom you've been given. Others will encourage his flock with love. Some will raise babies to know the kiss of Jesus while some will raise teams of integrity in the workplace. Regardless of where your life takes you, Jesus has taken hold of you for a purpose.

Turn to Ephesians 1:17-21. What is Paul's prayer for these believers? It's First Place for Health's prayer for you too.

_____

_____

Now, read Philippians 3:13-14. What must we do as we progress forward?

_____

_____

Paul said we must forget what lies behind us and press on ahead. In other words, we mustn't get stuck on past failures or attempts at change but must expectantly trust that new life is ahead. If we're stuck in the past, we can't lunge towards our future. And lunge we must.

Even though Philippians is called the letter of joy, Paul pulls no punches in the next verses as he talks about what gets in the way of our lunging. Read verses 17-21. Who brought Paul to tears?

Paul wept over those who lived in denial of the power of Christ. Their god is their stomach and they're proud of things that bring shame. Even to the end of his days, he tried to show there was a better way. I was one of those he wept for. My god was my appetite, and I boasted in what truthfully brought me shame. But then came the hope of change.

Read Philippians 4:11-13. How can we learn the secret of appetites and wants?

The secret is in the learning, and the learning is steeped in the strength of Christ. You have committed the past months to going deeper in the knowledge and the truth of living Beyond Free. Our Lord is so proud of you and will surely strengthen you as you spread your wings and freely fly.

My Lord, I want to know Your secrets--when being full or famished feels the same as long as I have You. Take me to this secret place and teach me this wonderful content-ment. I worship only You. Amen.

—— DAY 5: REVIVE
Oh Lord, refresh and renew me. Revive me according to your Word. Amen

I love the word revival. It used to conjure strange images in my mind of white tents and people acting crazy...but no more. For the past ten years I've studied great awakenings throughout the centuries, and they all begin with one simple concept—a refreshing and renewal between the Lord God and his beloved. It's not strange, nor is it conjured drama to revive in the Lord—it's essential. As a matter of fact, I believe if we're not hungry for personal revival, we may fall into the rut of religion and duty rather than power and hope.

Several years ago, I was reading through the Psalms and I came across one that impacted me greatly. It's the longest psalm in the Bible and according to one translation, the word revive is used ten times!

Please turn to Psalm 119. Although it contains many verses, read the Psalm through without interruption. What theme do you see arising again and again?

_____

_____

Psalm 119 was written in praise to the goodness of God's Word and the hope we have for it to revive us in times of need. Look at Psalm 119:2. Whom did the psalmist say is blessed?

_____

_____

Now look at verses 9-16. What are some of the actions we take to let the word impact and protect us?

Vs. 9: _____

Vs. 10: _____

Vs. 11: _____

Vs. 13: _____

Vs. 16: _____

I love this psalm because it takes us through the gamut of emotions that any lover of God authentically experiences. If we're not honest about our need for God's reviving touch, there's a good chance we're missing the point completely. The psalmist's emotions rival a roller coaster at any theme park you can mention. He's up and he's down.

Read verses 36 and 37 below.
"Turn my heart towards your statues and not towards selfish gain. Turn my eyes away from worthless things; preserve my life according to your word."

What are some of the worthless things you long for God to turn you away from?

_____

_____

Turn to verses 105-112. What is the visual the psalmist gave us of God's Word (vs. 105) and what is our commitment to its truth (vs. 111-112)?

How does the psalmist show his love for God in verses 145-148? How can we model this love in our own lives?

When I don't sleep, my mind tends to spiral, and if I'm not careful, I may end up in a rabbit hole of worry. At dawn and during the night watches the psalmist was crying out for help. This has become my model. Instead of worry I make my sleepless time-frames a sanctuary for prayer. Is there a time of day or night you feel closest to the Lord? Is there a time you feel more reflective, frightened, or needy?

The last verses in this beautiful psalm give us a breath prayer that covers anything that overwhelms us. Let's say them to ourselves.

> "May my lips overflow with praise, for you teach me your decrees. May my tongue sing of your word, for all your commands are righteous. May your hand be ready to help me, for I have chosen your precepts." (Psalm 119:171-173)

Lord God, as we seek to live free, thank You for the renewal that we can find in Your Word. Amen.

—— DAY 6: REFLECTION AND APPLICATION

Jesus, I trust You today, no matter how I feel or what presents itself as an obstacle. Remind me that You have overcome anything that seems to overcome me. Amen.

Yesterday we studied Psalm 119, the longest psalm in the Bible. One of the things that strikes me about this psalm is the timeframes the psalmist mentioned that he prayed and gave praise. He men-tioned midnight, early morning, and night watches as times he prayed. One of the most interesting things he noted was in verse 164. He said "Seven times a day I praise you...." Why seven times? We could assume he knew seven was God's number of completion, but truthfully, we don't know.

It's evident that the psalmist took praise and prayer seriously, and so should we. So, I'm offering what I'll call the Psalm 119 Challenge. Set your alarm for seven times throughout the day and when it goes off, simply thank God for his word and the gift of his love. Focusing our mind directly on him seven times throughout the day (and hopefully more) will change our outlook and revive our hearts.

Jesus, seven times a day I will intentionally praise You. Let my lips offer a tangible sacrifice of love. Amen.

—— DAY 7: REFLECTION AND APPLICATION
Holy Spirit, bring to remembrance everything You have taught me over the past ten weeks. Let it soak into my spirit like a healing balm. Amen.

Look back over the titles of each of our weeks. Reflect on one of the chapters that especially resonated with you, and leaf through the pages of that chapter. Pray the Holy Spirit will bring to remembrance what you studied—and ask him to change you profoundly from the time you've offered to study and learn.

- Freedom Versus Dieting
- My Personal Exodus
- Battle Scars
- Breaking Generational Cycles
- Planting New Fields
- Time for Harvest
- Teach Us to Pray
- God on the Move
- What's Going On?
- Living Beyond Free

Dearest Lord, freedom is never free. My freedom cost You everything, and I joyfully and mightily take hold of it. I pray to never let go. Amen.

Notes
1. I wrote a book called Spirit Hunger that exposes our deep longing to connect with God.
2. Geneen Roth, Breaking Free from Compulsive Eating (New York: Plume/Penguin, 2003), 7-8.

WEEK ELEVEN: REVIEW AND REFLECT

To help you shape your short victory celebration testimony, work through the following questions in your prayer journal, one on each day leading up to your group's celebration:

DAY ONE: List some of the benefits you have gained by allowing the Lord to transform your life through this twelve-week First Place for Health session. Be mindful that He has been active in all four aspects of your being, so list benefits you have received in the physical, mental, emotional and spiritual realms.

DAY TWO: In what ways have you most significantly changed mentally? Have you seen a shift in the ways you think about yourself, food, your relationships, or God? How has Scripture memory been a part of these shifts?

DAY THREE: In what ways have you most significantly changed emotionally? Have you begun to identify how your feelings influence your relationship to food and exercise? What are you doing to stay aware of your emotions, both positive and negative?

DAY FOUR: In what ways have you most significantly changed spiritually? How has your relationship with God deepened? How has drawing closer to Him made a difference in the other three areas of your life?

DAY FIVE: In what ways have you most significantly changed physically? Have you met or exceeded your weight/measurement goals? How has your health improved during the past twelve weeks?

DAY SIX: Was there one person in your First Place for Health group who was particularly encouraging to you? How did their kindness make a difference in your First Place for Health journey?

DAY SEVEN: Summarize the previous six questions into a one-page testimony, or "faith story," to share at your group's victory celebration.

May the example of the biblical characters we studied continue to inspire you to build strength into your life mentally, emotionally, and spiritually. May our strong Lord guide and direct all your days ahead as you choose to make Him first place in your life!

WEEK TWELVE: A TIME TO CELEBRATE!

Join your group in celebrating the benefits you have gained, the shift in the way you see yourself, how your relationship with God has changed, and the improvement in your health. Spend time celebrating your group and the encouragement you have experienced through each other. Celebrate!

LEADER DISCUSSION GUIDE

For in-depth information, guidance and helpful tips about leading a successful First Place for Health group, spend time studying the *My Place for Leadership* book. In it, you will find valuable answers to most of your questions, as well as personal insights from many First Place for Health group leaders.

For the group meetings in this session, be sure to read and consider each week's discussion topics several days before the meeting—some questions and activities require supplies and/or planning to complete. Also, if you are leading a large group, plan to break into smaller groups for discussion and then come together as a large group to share your answers and responses. Make sure to appoint a capable leader for each small group so that discussions stay focused and on track (and be sure each group records their answers!).

—— WEEK ONE: FREEDOM VERSUS DIETING

On Day One we saw it's not about willpower—because over time complacency, deception, and defeat creep in. How is the pursuit of freedom much deeper than tips on how to increase our willpower? (Note to leaders: willpower isn't a bad thing—it leads to self-control, which is a fruit of the spirit. In this section we're stating that our will alone doesn't have the power to defeat our struggles. Only the power of God united with our will to change brings lasting results.)

Most of us have tried diets and failed. We may have had temporary success with weight loss but eventually landed right back where we started...or worse! On Day Two we mention three ways dieting is different from true freedom. Which of the following do you struggle with or long to understand more deeply? Discuss why these may be hard to grasp.

- Dieting is temporary; freedom is a gift for life.
- Dieting is carnal; freedom is spiritual.
- Diets are band aids; freedom is life change.

On Day Three we looked at the lure of slavery. Why is slavery, at times, easier than the pursuit of freedom? In Exodus 15:26 God says, "I, the Lord, am your healer." Ask group members how this encourages them as they start (or continue) the journey towards living *Beyond Free*.

—— WEEK TWO: MY PERSONAL EXODUS

Discuss with your group the meaning of spiritual oppression. If it covers anything that keeps us from growing in our full identity with God, how has food and weight been oppressive?

On Day Two we studied the idea that freedom requires sacrifice and the belief that life can be different. We also observed the hard fact that sometimes when we decide to do something about slavery, the bondage tightens its grip. What kinds of sacrifice may be necessary to truly moves towards freedom? If things feel worse as we begin to pursue freedom, how can we be assured God doesn't promise things he isn't prepared to deliver?

Imagine being an Israelite during the plagues and the Passover. What a stressful period! On Day Three we discussed how in his directions regarding the Passover meal God said to leave no leftovers and be ready to move. This was a measure of trust as it meant they had to solely depend on God for what was next. To be free, we must to the same. What does that look like practically—in our day-to-day?

The title of Day Four is Waking the Miracle. It's tempting to think miracles of healing and hope just happen but there's always a period of waking—transitioning from one mindset to the next. When the Israelites were faced with crisis as they watched their enemy riding after them in the sea, they quickly forgot that God parted the waters for them. As a group discuss the tension between asking God for miracles and experiencing the emotions of fear and panic or the belief that things will never change.

—— WEEK THREE: BATTLE SCARS

How is understanding the enemy's schematic for our lives just as important as putting on the armor God's given us to fight?

We learned that the enemy draws his schematic based on the following:

- Identity: Who God created us to be
- Purpose: What God created us to do
- Provision: How we acknowledge who God has created us to be and accomplish what he's called us to do

Knowing this, how can we be prepared for the schematic unique to our lives? Discuss where each group member feels the most vulnerable.

On Day One we looked at what Dr. Charles Stanley calls a "point of access" in which the enemy pushes in. We followed that point of access in Paul's life and found it to be pride. According to the book of Acts, Jesus used three blind days to change Paul's schematic. Talk about what the points of access are in our lives and how God has changed our schematic in the past—or is in the state of changing it now.

We looked at Daniel's life on Day Three and saw there were many point of entry moments in which he acted wisely or faithfully—changing the course of his life and the lives of those around him for good. Instead of giving the enemy access, he defeated him from the start. Talk about these point of entry moment actions and decide which inspire you based on what you're facing now:

1. Make up your mind.
2. Believe you can be successful even if you're not sure how. Ask for the help of those you trust. Strength rises on the backs of those who believe.
3. Stay on your knees no matter who is watching. When the enemy shuts the door, fling the windows open wide.
4. Tested faith brings rugged assurance. Not only in the one tested, but those who watch the test.

As we continued to look at Daniel on Day Four, we studied the symbolic horn that boastfully tried to drown out the worship of the Messiah King. We noted the words of Carole Lewis (First Place national director emeritus): "The voice of the Holy Spirit is kind while the voice of the devil is mean." Share what this obnoxious voice sounds like to each member and how the Holy Spirit's voice differs in its tone.

—— WEEK FOUR: BREAKING GENERATIONAL CYCLES

On Day One we examined patterns of destructive behavior in our families originating in the generations before us. Going back one to two generations (parents and grandparents), what kind of destructive patterns do you see? Ask group members how these patterns have impacted their lives.

We noted in Ezekiel 18 a child will not share the guilt of a parent. Even so, a common theme in Jesus's day (and ours) was to figure out and blame someone for struggles. According to John 9, ask group members what the purpose of pain and hardship is and how that is a comfort when they experience trouble from their past.

On Day Two we note that forgiveness of our past offenders isn't an option; it's a command. Talk about how Joseph (Genesis 45:1-8) acknowledged the pain he endured at his brothers' hands. He broke the power of his generational curse by forgiving his painful past, not by ignoring or excusing it. Gently ask group members if there's someone they need to forgive to break a generational curse in their lives.

How does the story of Elisha and King Joash (Day 3) represent a bigger story of faith in what God can do when we trust him? Share how we can "bang our arrows" for the more God wants to give us as we trust.

How can we tell the difference between speech motivated by the curses of Satan or the comfort of God (Day Five)? Share why new names matter (like the new name God gave Peter). Ask members to share what new name God might give to them, even if they aren't fully living it yet!

—— WEEK FIVE: PLANTING NEW FIELDS

How do Paul's words in Galatians 6 lay the groundwork for seed-sowing in our lives? What do we sow towards life and what is sown towards destruction?

On Day One the author mentions the difference between Spirit Seeds and Flesh Seeds. Ask members how these seeds are evident in their behaviors and choices. Then go on to share about the specific seeds they have offered to the Lord for sowing. Be sure to discuss how these seeds are different from dieting.

Day Three covers how a bully thinks. We learn that:

1. A bully sees us as weak.
2. A bully assumes a posture of dominance.
3. Bullies are afraid to lose power, so they hurt those they feel they can control.

Ask your group to share which scriptures noted speak loudest to the bully that pushes them around the most.

Secrets are also exposed on Day Three. Many of us don't realize the ways we hide our eating habits or behaviors. Discuss how sowing seeds to secrets can expose these behaviors as they lose their power.

On Day Four we notice how Paul mentioned we shouldn't sow seeds—reluctantly or under compulsion. As a group, can you name times that trying to behave "right" with food felt more compulsive than productive? Why? Why is it so important to sow abundantly not sparingly?

Unlike dieting, share how seed sowing is an act of worship.

—— WEEK SIX: TIME FOR HARVEST

Start by discussing the author's comment on Day One: "We need to quit thinking obedience is optional and start viewing it as essential." Ask members to authentically share how they've been viewing obedience.

We also looked at things we start and stop (Day One). These are the things we plant and sow that never come to a harvest. This may not be exclusive to behaviors with food and may include things we've tried to pursue: dreams, jobs, relationships. Are there fields in our lives we've never harvested because harvest is hard?

On Day Three we studied how in biblical times vineyards were protected by a hedge. Spiritually, a hedge is the promise of God's protection for those who love and walk with him. Discuss which of the hedges mentioned in our lesson empower the group the most. Why?

We also looked at the concept of fire built in the vineyard before a harvest (Day Three). Why do you think before we reap the greatest blessings "Every power in hell, insect, and fowl bird wants to lodge in our branches"?

Name a harvest blocker you see in your life right now. Discuss how can you remove it so it doesn't keep you from your reward.

—— WEEK SEVEN: TEACH US TO PRAY

On Day One Jesus explains why it's not always easy to pray. Our spirits are willing, but our flesh is weak. In the Prayer of Surrender we see how things we're told to focus on (Philippians 4:8) differ from their fake counterparts. Talk about which words jump off that chart as things we need to surrender.

Discuss which of these statements from Day Two get in the way of Healing Prayer:

1. We pray, and nothing seems to change.
2. We're in the way of God's next steps.
3. We're in a hurry to see results and when we don't, we lose faith.

On Day Three the Prayer of Authority takes charge of the situation and puts things in place. How do we view Jesus's words from Luke 9:1-12? Are we authority takers in prayer or merely reactive?

We need to practice authority in both mundane activities as well as big challenges. Talk about why that's not always easy. As a group, share some of your Prayer Commands from Day Three.

Does the concept of unceasing prayer seem overwhelming? Share ideas and thoughts on how we can keep our minds centered on Jesus and enjoy this invitation given by the apostle Paul. How does the notion of breath prayer help?

On Day Five we looked at prayer for territory and blessing while studying the prayer uttered by a man named Jabez. His prayers centered on:

- Blessings
- Influence (territory)
- Presence
- Protection

Which of these focused areas get you most excited? Which do you need the most right now?

—— WEEK EIGHT: GOD ON THE MOVE

Why is the apostle Paul's concept of making our bodies our slave, rather than us being our body's slave so important (1 Cor. 9:24-27)? What does being a slave to our body feel like?

For fun, ask your group what they think of Mary's fitness aptitude on Day One? (Jesus's mother).

Day Two focused on rebuilding the temple and the words from the prophet Haggai to "consider your ways." How is this statement the perfect place to begin when considering rebuilding our bodies?

The author introduced us to a man named Zerubbabel on Day Two. What strikes you about this man and why is he a good model for us?

On Day Three we studied how Paul says we must give ourselves fully to the work of the Lord. How can going for a walk or exercising be as holy as serving?

Ask group members to share their thoughts on what a perfect body would look like (Day Three). Then reflect on the question, "Are there old plans and strategies for dealing with your weight that no longer work?" If so, what new ideas can you use for results rather than predictable failure?

—— WEEK NINE: WHAT'S GOING ON

This week we studied the strategies God uses to bring growth in our lives: disciplining, sifting, and pruning. Ask your group about their impression of this truth on

Day One: DISCIPLINING = PROTECTION. How is this comforting rather than punishing?

On Day Two the author explained that as we mature in God's discipline, He brings checkpoints or tests, where we can show what we know. Why do pliable people perform better on these tests? What happens when we're rigid and refuse to learn?

Day Three established that discipline is from the Father, but sifting is from the enemy. If discipline is meant to protect us, sifting is meant to rattle us. Think about the sifting examples of Peter and Job. What were the outcomes of these seasons of sifting? Ask members to share if they are in a season like this or if they can recall a time of sifting. How did it feel different than a season of disciplining? Why must we lean into God during times of sifting rather than shout forceful demands for blessing and outcomes?

Day Four talks about pruning and the need for God to cut away branches that don't bear fruit. From the list below, where do you see the need to be pruned?

- Priorities that need to be rearranged
- Relationships that need to change or end
- Busyness that isn't accomplishing what matters most
- Dependencies or attachments that we're ready to grow out of

On Day Five we talked about principles of abiding. Remember, abiding is not serving. Have members share if they are abiders or doers. According to what we learned in Day Five, how can we truly abide?

—— WEEK TEN: LIVING BEYOND FREE

Ask members to turn to the quote by Geneen Roth on Day One. She talks about food being the glue that held her life together between hungers. Share your own experiences with hunger and ask the group to share too. Do we understand it? Do we ignore it? Do we eat out of habit or body hunger—or is some of what we feel actually a Spirit Hunger?

Jesus spoke of food that perishes and food that endures to eternal life. What do you think the difference is (Day One)?

Discuss why you think it's important that in Psalm 23 the Lord prepares a table for us in the presence of our enemies—not in a backroom or basement (Day Two).

Mary of Bethany was "all in" when she lavishly anointed Jesus's head with costly perfume (Day Three). His words to her and the crowd watching still ring true to us today:

1.   She's done a good deed.
2.   She's done what she could.
3.   Her act is now a memory of love towards Jesus.

Which of these statements would you most like to hear Jesus say to you today? Why?

On Day Four, think about Paul's comment "to take hold of that for which Jesus took hold of me." Why did Jesus take hold of you? What do you think were some of his purposes?

Day Five showed how the psalmist spoke repeatedly in Psalm 119 of a personal revival. He had certain timeframes he set apart to praise the Lord (midnight, in the night watches, seven times a day). Share times you can set apart to stop and praise. How will this transform your days?

FIRST PLACE FOR HEALTH
JUMP START MENUS

This week of recipes is based on approximately 1,300 to 1,400 calories per day, allowing for snack or dessert options up to 200 calories per day. All recipe and menu nutritional information was determined using the MasterCook software, a program that accesses a database containing more than 6,000 food items prepared using the United States Department of Agriculture (USDA) publications and information from food manufacturers. As with any nutritional program, MasterCook calculates the nutritional values of the recipes based on ingredients. Nutrition may vary due to how the food is prepared, where the food comes from, soil content, season, ripeness, processing and method of preparation. For these reasons, please use the recipes and menu plans as approximate guides. As always, consult your physician and/or a registered dietitian before starting a weight-loss program.

For those who need more calories,

add the following to the 1,400–1,500 calorie plan:

1,500-1,600 calories:	1 oz.-eq of protein, 1 oz.-eq. grains, ½ cup vegetables, 1 tsp. healthy oils
1,700-1,800 calories:	1½ oz.-eq. of protein, 2 oz.-eq. grains, 1 cup of vegetables, 1 tsp. healthy oils
1,900-2,000 calories:	2 oz.-eq. of protein, 2 oz.-eq. of grains, 1 cup vegetables, ½ cup fruit, 1 tsp. healthy oils
2,100-2,200 calories:	3 oz.-eq. of protein, 3 oz.-eq. grains, 1½ cup vegetables, ½ cup fruit, 2 tsp. healthy oils
2,300-2,400 calories:	4 oz.-eq. of protein, 4 oz.-eq. of grains, 2 cups vegetables 3 cups frit, 3 tsp. healthy oils

DAY 1 | BREAKFAST

Peanut Butter Smoothie

½ cup low-fat milk
⅓ cup nonfat plain Greek yogurt
1 cup baby spinach
1 cup frozen banana slices (about 1 medium banana)
½ cup frozen strawberries
1 tbsp. natural peanut butter
1-2 tsp. honey (optional)

Add milk and yogurt to a blender, then add spinach, banana, strawberries, peanut butter and honey (if using); blend until smooth. Serves 1.

Nutritional Information: 327 calories; 10.2 g total fat; 10 mg cholesterol; 160 mg sodium. 53.9 g carbohydrates; 18.1 g protein

Live It Tracker: 1 1/2 cups fruit, 1/2 cup dairy, 1 oz.-eq protein, 1/2 tsp. healthy oil

Creamy Avocado & White Bean Wrap

2 tbsp. cider vinegar

1 tbsp. canola oil

2 tsp. finely chopped canned chipotle chile in adobo sauce

¼ tsp. salt

2 cups shredded red cabbage

1 medium carrot, shredded

¼ cup chopped fresh cilantro

1 15-ounce can white beans, rinsed

1 ripe avocado

½ cup shredded sharp Cheddar cheese

2 tbsp. minced red onion

4 8-10-inch whole-wheat wraps or tortillas

Whisk vinegar, oil, chipotle chile and salt in a medium bowl. Add cabbage, carrot and cilantro; toss to combine. Mash beans and avocado in another medium bowl with a potato masher or fork. Stir in cheese and onion. To assemble the wraps, spread about 1/2 cup of the bean-avocado mixture onto a wrap (or tortilla) and top with about 2/3 cup of the cabbage-carrot slaw. Roll up. Repeat with remaining ingredients. Cut the wraps in half to serve, if desired.

Nutritional Information: 346 calories; 17 g total fat; 14 mg cholesterol; 465 mg sodium. 44.2 g carbohydrates; 11.8 g protein

Live It Tracker: 2 oz.-eq. grain, 1 cup vegetable, 1 tsp. healthy oil

Beef & Bean Sloppy Joes

1 tbsp. extra-virgin olive oil
12 ounces lean ground beef
1 cup no-salt-added black beans, rinsed
1 cup chopped onion
2 tsp. chile powder
½ tsp. garlic powder
½ tsp. onion powder
Pinch of cayenne pepper
1 cup no-salt-added tomato sauce
3 tbsp. ketchup
1 tbsp. reduced-sodium Worcestershire sauce
2 tsp. spicy brown mustard
1 tsp. light brown sugar
4 whole-wheat hamburger buns, split and toasted

Heat oil in a large nonstick skillet over medium-high heat. Add beef and cook, breaking it up with a spoon, until lightly browned, but not completely cooked through, 3 to 4 minutes. Using a slotted spoon, transfer the beef to a medium bowl, reserving drippings in the pan. Add beans and onion to the pan. Cook, stirring often, until the onion is softened, about 5 minutes. Add chile powder, garlic powder, onion powder and cayenne. Cook, stirring constantly, until fragrant, about 30 seconds. Stir in tomato sauce, ketchup, Worcestershire, mustard and brown sugar. Return the beef to the pan. Bring to a simmer and cook, stirring often, until the beef is just cooked through and the sauce has thickened slightly, about 5 minutes. Serve on buns. Serves 4.

Nutrition information: 411 calories; 15 g total fat; 55 mg cholesterol; 537 mg sodium. 43.8 g carbohydrates; 25.8 g protein

Live It Tracker: 3 oz.-eq. protein, 2 oz.-eq. grain, 1/2 cups vegetable

Blueberry Almond Overnight Oats

⅓ cup oats
½ cup milk
1 tsp. chia seeds
½ tbsp. maple syrup
1 tsp. vanilla extract
2 tbsp. slivered almonds
½ medium banana, sliced
⅓ cup blueberries

In an airtight container, mix oats, milk, chia seeds, maple syrup, and vanilla. Seal the container and place in the fridge overnight. In the morning, stir oats and top with slivered almonds, sliced banana, and blueberries. Serves 1.

Nutritional Information: 341 Calories; 9g Fat; 97mg Sodium; 54g Carbohydrates; 9g Protein

Live It Tracker: 1 oz.-eq. protein, 1 oz.-eq. grain, 1 cup fruit, 1 tsp. healthy oil

Veggie & Hummus Sandwich

2 slices whole-grain bread

3 tbsp. hummus

¼ avocado, mashed

½ cup mixed salad greens

¼ medium red bell pepper, sliced

¼ cup sliced cucumber

¼ cup shredded carrot

Spread one slice of bread with hummus and the other with avocado. Fill the sandwich with greens, bell pepper, cucumber and carrot. Slice in half and serve. Serves 1

Nutritional Information: 325 calories; 14.3 g total fat; 407 mg sodium. 39.7 g carbohydrates; 12.8 g protein

Live It Tracker: 1/2 oz.-eq. protein, 1 1/2 oz.-eq. grain, 1 cup vegetable, 1 tsp. healthy oil

One-Pan Pesto Chicken and Veggies

2 tbsp. olive oil

1 lb. chicken thighs boneless and skinless, sliced into strips

1/3 cup sun-dried tomatoes drained of oil, chopped

1 lb. asparagus trimmed and cut in half

1/4 cup basil pesto

1 cup cherry tomatoes, halved

Heat a large skillet on medium heat, add 2 tbsp. olive oil, sliced chicken thighs. Season chicken generously with salt. Add half of chopped sun-dried tomatoes and cook on medium heat for 5-10 minutes, turning a couple of times, until the chicken is completely cooked through. Remove the chicken and sun-dried tomatoes from the skillet, leaving oil. Add asparagus, seasoned with salt and remaining half of sun-dried tomatoes. Cook on medium heat for 5-10 minutes until the asparagus is cooked through. Remove asparagus to serving plate. Add chicken back to the skillet. Add pesto and stir to coat on low-medium heat until chicken is reheated, 1 or 2 minutes. Remove from heat. Add halved cherry to-matoes and mix with the pesto and the chicken. Add chicken and tomatoes to the serving plate with asparagus. Serves 4.

Nutrition information: 423 calories; 32g fat; 23g protein; 261mg sodium

Live It Tracker: 3 oz.-eq. protein, 1 cup vegetables

Breakfast Egg Muffins

cooking spray
6 eggs
salt and pepper to taste
½ cup cooked chopped spinach, excess water removed
⅓ cup cooked bacon, crumbled
⅓ cup shredded cheddar cheese
diced tomatoes and chopped parsley optional garnish

Preheat the oven to 375o degrees. Coat 6 cups of a muffin tin with cooking spray or line with paper liners. Crack the eggs into a large bowl. Whisk to blend the eggs until smooth. Add the spinach, bacon and cheese to the egg mixture and stir to combine. Divide the egg mixture evenly among the muffin cups. Bake for 15-18 minutes or until eggs are set. Serve immediately or store in the refrigerator until ready to eat. Top with diced tomatoes and parsley, if desired. Serves 6.

Nutritional Information: 129 calories; 10g fat; 220mg sodium; 1g carbohydrate; 0.8g protein

Live It Tracker: 1 oz.-eq. protein

Mason Jar Power Salad with Tuna

3 cups bite-sized pieces chopped kale
2 tbsp. honey-mustard vinaigrette
1 2.5-ounce pouch tuna in water
½ cup rinsed canned chickpeas
1 carrot, peeled and shredded

Toss kale and dressing in a bowl, then transfer to a 1-quart mason jar. Top with tuna, chickpeas and carrot. Screw lid onto the jar and refrigerate for up to 2 days. To serve, empty the jar contents into a bowl and toss to combine the salad ingredients with the dressed kale. Serves 1.

Nutritional Information: 430 calories; 22.7g total fat; 496mg sodium. 30.1 carbohydrates; 26.4g protein

Live It Tracker: 2 1/2 oz.-eq. protein, 1 oz.-eq. grain; 1 cup vegetable

Cheesy Taco Stuffed Zucchini

3 medium sized zucchini, cut in half lengthwise
1/2 lb. lean ground beef
1/3 cup diced onion
1 clove garlic, grated
1 tsp. chili powder
1 tsp. ground cumin
1/4 tsp. oregano
Kosher salt and fresh ground black pepper to taste
4 ounce can diced green chiles
1 1/2 cups cauliflower rice (fresh or frozen)
3/4 cup salsa, divided
1/2 cup shredded Colby jack cheese
1/2 cup chopped tomatoes
Cilantro for garnish

Preheat oven to 400°F. Place 1/4 cup of salsa in the bottom of a large baking dish. Use a small spoon or metal 1/2 tsp. measuring spoon to hollow out the center of the zucchini halves then place them cut side up in the prepared baking dish. Leave approximately 1/4-inch thick shell on each half. Heat a large skillet over medium-high heat and spray with cooking oil. Add the onion and cook for approximately two minutes. Add the ground beef to the skillet and break it up into small crumbles as it cooks. Cook until the beef is no longer pink then add in the garlic, spices, green chiles, cauliflower rice and remaining 1/2 cup of salsa. Taste for seasoning. Mix everything together until combined and cook until heated through, about 3-5 minutes. Divide the taco filling equally into the hollowed zucchini boats, pressing it in firmly. Top with shredded cheese then cover with foil and bake 25-35 minutes or until cheese is melted and zucchini is cooked through. Top with cilantro and serve with extra salsa on the side. Serves 3.

Nutritional Information: 367 calories; 24.8 g total fat; 7.7 g saturated fat; 68 mg cholesterol; 659 mg sodium; 14.3 g carbohydrates; 24.8 g protein

Live It Tracker: 3 oz.-eq.- protein, 1 cup vegetable

Microwave Egg and Spinach Breakfast Sandwich

1 Everything Bagel Thin
1 Large Egg
fresh spinach leaves
2 tbsp whipped cream cheese
2 slices tomato
2 slices avocado
kosher salt
hot sauce

Toast bagel thin in the toaster. In a small bowl add egg and spinach leaves, season with kosher salt. Place in microwave for 1 minute 30 seconds. Spread cream cheese on toasted bagel thin and add slices of tomato. Spoon egg out of bowl and place on top of cheese and tomato, top with avocado. Season with more salt and hot sauce, if desired. Serves 1.

Nutritional Information: 302 calories; 12.7 g total fat; 3.2 g saturated fat; 191 mg cholesterol; 646 mg sodium. 886 mg potassium; 29.7 g carbohydrates; 6 g fiber; 3 g sugar; 18.5 g protein

Live It Tracker: 1 oz.-eq. protein; 1 1/2 oz.-eq. grain, 1/2 cup vegetable

Ravioli & Vegetable Soup

1 tbsp. extra-virgin olive oil
2 cups frozen bell pepper and onion mix, thawed and diced
2 cloves garlic, minced
1/4 tsp. crushed red pepper, (optional)
1 28-ounce can crushed fire-roasted tomatoes
1 15-ounce can vegetable broth or reduced-sodium chicken broth
1½ cups hot water
1 tsp. dried basil
1 6- to 9-ounce package fresh or frozen cheese (or meat) ravioli
2 cups diced zucchini, (about 2 medium)
Freshly ground pepper to taste

Heat oil in a large saucepan or Dutch oven over medium heat. Add pepper-onion mix, garlic and crushed red pepper (if using) and cook, stirring, for 1 minute. Add tomatoes, broth, water and basil and bring to a rolling boil over high heat. Add ravioli and cook for three minutes less than the package directions. Add zucchini; return to a boil. Cook until the zucchini is crisp-tender, about 3 minutes. Season with pepper. Serves 4.

Nutritional Information: 261 calories; 8.3 g total fat; 28 mg cholesterol; 354 mg sodium. 32.6 g carbohydrates; 10.6 g protein

Live It Tracker: 1 oz.-eq. grain, 1 cup vegetable

DAY 4 | DINNER

Hearty Tomato Soup with Beans & Greens

2 14-ounce cans low-sodium hearty-style tomato soup
1 tbsp. olive oil
3 cups chopped kale
1 tsp. minced garlic
⅛ tsp. crushed red pepper (optional)
1 14 ounce can no-salt-added cannellini beans, rinsed
¼ cup grated Parmesan cheese

Heat soup in a medium saucepan according to package directions; simmer over low heat as you prepare kale. Heat oil in a large skillet over medium heat. Add kale and cook, stirring, until wilted, one to two minutes. Stir in garlic and crushed red pepper, if using, and cook for 30 seconds. Stir the greens and beans into the soup and simmer until the beans are heated through, two to three minutes. Divide the soup among four bowls. Serve topped with Parmesan. Serves 4.

Nutritional Information: 200 calories; 5.8 g total fat; 4 mg cholesterol; 355 mg sodium. 29 g carbohydrates; 8.6 g protein

Live It Tracker: 1 oz.-eq. protein, 1/2 oz.-eq. grain, 1/2 cup vegetable

Chocolate Banana Oatmeal Smoothie Bowl

½ cup old-fashioned oats
1 tbsp chia seeds
2 tbsp unsweetened cocoa
1 cup fat-free milk
1 medium-size ripe banana, frozen

The night before, add all the ingredients except the frozen banana to the bowl of your blender and stir to combine. Cover and place in the fridge for at least 3 hours, preferably overnight. When ready to eat, add the frozen banana and blend on high until oats are fully broken down and a smooth and creamy consistency is reached, adding more milk if the smoothie is too thick. Transfer it to a bowl, garnish with toppings of choice. Serves 1.

Nutritional Information: 302 calories; 9.3g fat, 203.7mg sodium, 43.2mg carbohydrate; 11.8g protein

Live It Tracker: 1 oz.-eq. grain, 1 cup dairy, 1 cup fruit

Avocado Ranch Chicken Salad

1 ripe avocado, halved and pitted
⅓ cup ranch dressing
2 tablespoons chopped pickled jalapeño
1 tbsp. white-wine vinegar
¼ tsp. salt
¼ tsp. ground pepper
3 cups shredded or chopped cooked chicken
½ cup diced celery
¼ cup diced red onion

Scoop avocado into a food processor. Add ranch dressing, pickled jalapeño, vinegar, salt and pepper. Pulse until smooth. Transfer to a medium bowl. Add chicken, celery and red onion; mix with a rubber spatula. Serve at room temperature or refrigerate until cold, about 2 hours. Serves 6.

Nutritional Information: calories 361 calories; 23.1 g total fat; 117 mg cholesterol; 350 mg sodium. 4.7 g carbohydrates; 32.5 g protein

Live It Tracker: 3 oz.-eq. protein, 1/2 cup vegetable, 1 tsp. healthy oil

Roasted Parmesan Chicken and Tomatoes

4 boneless, skinless chicken breast fillets
Kosher salt and black pepper
1/4 cup panko breadcrumbs
1/4 cup grated Parmesan
1 tbsp. olive oil
1 tbsp. chopped fresh flat-leaf parsley
1 chopped garlic clove
1 tsp. Dijon mustard
1 lb.. Campari Tomatoes

Preheat oven to 450°F. Arrange chicken breast fillets on an aluminum foil-lined baking sheet. Season with kosher salt and black pepper. Stir together panko breadcrumbs, grated Parmesan, olive oil, chopped parsley, and chopped garlic clove. Spread Dijon mustard on each chicken breast. Sprinkle with breadcrumb mixture. Arrange Campari tomatoes around chicken. Bake until chicken is just cooked through, 14 to 16 minutes. Serves 4.

Nutritional Information: 345 calories; 11.7 g total fat; 2.3 g saturated fat; 86 mg cholesterol; 517 mg sodium; 24.3 g carbohydrates; 35.7 g protein

Live It Tracker: 3 oz.-eq. protein, 1 cup vegetable

Baked Eggs with Spinach and Tomato

2 tbsp. olive oil

1 medium onion

5 oz. fresh baby spinach

1 14-ounce can whole tomatoes

1 tsp. ground cumin

1 tsp. salt

1 tsp. freshly ground pepper

½ tsp. sweet paprika

2 tsp. hot sauce

4 large eggs

¼ cup crumbled feta

Preheat oven to 400 degrees F. Meanwhile, in a medium saucepan, heat oil over medium-high heat. Add onion and sauté until soft, about five minutes. Add spinach and sauté until just wilted, about two minutes. Remove from heat. In a medium bowl, stir together tomatoes, cumin, salt, pepper, paprika, and, if desired, hot sauce. Add onion-spinach mixture and stir to combine. Divide among 4 oiled 10-ounce ramekins. Crack an egg into the center of each ramekin, then sprinkle on feta. Bake until whites are set but yolks remain soft, 12 to 15 minutes. Serves 4.

Nutritional Information:344 calories; 20.3 g total fat; 3.7 g saturated fat; 372 mg cholesterol; 653 mg sodium; 20.6 g carbohydrates; 21.4 g protein

Live It Tracker: 2 oz.-eq. protein, 1 cups vegetable, 1 tsp. oil

DAY 6 | LUNCH

Zesty Mediterranean Quinoa Salad

3 cups cooked quinoa
2 medium cucumbers, chopped
1 pint cherry tomatoes, halved
½ red onion, finely chopped
½ avocado, chopped
½ cup crumbled feta
2 tbsp. freshly chopped parsley, plus more for garnish

FOR THE DRESSING
⅓ cup extra-virgin olive oil
¼ cup red wine vinegar
1 tsp. honey
1 clove garlic, minced
kosher salt
½ tsp. crushed red pepper flakes
1 tsp. oregano

In a large bowl combine quinoa, cucumber, tomatoes, onion, avocado, feta and parsley. Make dressing: In a medium bowl, combine olive oil, vinegar, honey and garlic. Season with salt, red pepper flakes and oregano and whisk until combined. Pour dressing over salad mixture and toss until salad is coated in dressing. Garnish with more parsley and serve. Serves 4.

Nutritional Information: 182 calories; 8 g total fat; 152 mg sodium; 21.4 g carbohydrates; 7.8 g protein

Live It Tracker: 1 ½ oz.-eq. grain, ½ oz.-eq. protein, ½ cup vegetable

Creamy Lemon Pasta with Shrimp

8 ounces whole-wheat fettuccine

1 tbsp. extra-virgin olive oil

12 ounces peeled and deveined raw shrimp (26-30 per lb.)

2 tbsp. unsalted butter

1 tbsp. finely chopped garlic

¼ tsp. crushed red pepper

4 cups loosely packed arugula

¼ cup plain yogurt

1 tsp. lemon zest

2 tbsp. lemon juice

¼ tsp. salt

⅓ cup grated Parmesan cheese, plus more for garnish

¼ cup thinly sliced fresh basil

Bring seven cups of water to a boil. Add fettuccine, stirring to separate the noodles. Cook until just tender, 7 to 9 minutes. Reserve 1/2 cup of the cooking water and drain. Meanwhile, heat oil in a large nonstick skillet over medium-high heat. Add shrimp and cook, stirring occasionally, until pink and curled, 2 to 3 minutes. Transfer the shrimp to a bowl. Add butter to the pan and reduce heat to medium. Add garlic and crushed red pepper; cook, stirring often, until the garlic is fragrant, about one minute. Add arugula and cook, stirring, until wilted, about one minute. Reduce heat to low. Add the fettuccine, yogurt, lemon zest and the reserved cooking water, 1/4 cup at a time, tossing well, until the fettuccine is fully coated and creamy. Add the shrimp, lemon juice and salt, tossing to coat the fettuccine. Remove from the heat and toss with Parmesan. Serve the fettuccine topped with basil and more Parmesan, if desired. Serves 4.

Nutritional Information: 403 calories; 13.9 g total fat; 160 mg cholesterol; 396 mg sodium. 45.5 g carbohydrates; 28.3 g protein

Live It Tracker: 2 ½ oz.-eq. protein, 2 oz.-eq. grain, 1 tsp. healthy oil

Sweet and Crunchy Yogurt Topping

Nonstick cooking spray
2 cups old-fashioned oats
¾ cup coarsely chopped walnuts and/or almonds
¼ cup packed brown sugar
2 tbsp. canola oil
⅛ tsp. salt
¼ tsp. ground cinnamon
10 cups plain fat-free yogurt

Preheat oven to 325 degrees F. Coat a 15x10x1-inch baking pan with nonstick cooking spray; set aside. In a large bowl, combine oats, nuts, brown sugar, oil, salt, and, if desired, cinnamon. Spread in an even layer in prepared baking pan. Bake about 25 minutes or until golden brown, stirring twice. Spread on a large piece of foil to cool. For each serving, spoon 1/2 cup of the yogurt into a parfait glass or dessert dish; sprinkle with 2 tbsp. of the oat mixture. Store oat mixture in an airtight container at room temperature for up to 3 weeks or freeze for up to 3 months. Serves 20.

Nutritional Information: 150 calories; 5 g total fat; 2 mg cholesterol; 110 mg sodium. 18.1 g carbohydrates; 8.7 g proteinLive It Tracker: 1/2 oz.-eq. grain,

1/2 cup dairy, 1/2 tsp. healthy oil

Taco Salad in a Jar

    2 tbsp. extra-virgin olive oil
    1 lb. ground turkey
    kosher salt
    1 tbsp. Taco Seasoning
    1 15-oz. can black beans, rinsed and warmed
    2 cup frozen corn, thawed and warmed
    1 head romaine, chopped
    1 cup shredded pepper Jack cheese
    1 cup diced tomatoes

In a large skillet, heat oil over medium-high heat. Add turkey and season with salt and taco seasoning. Cook, breaking up with the back of a wooden spoon or spatula, until deeply golden and cooked through, 8 to 10 minutes. Set aside and let cool 5 minutes. Among six mason jars, layer ground turkey, black beans, corn, romaine, cheese, and tomatoes. Keep cool. Serves 6.

Nutritional Information: 440 calories; 32g carbohydrate; 650mg sodium; 28g protein

Live It Tracker: 3 oz.-eq. protein, 1 cup vegetable; ⅔ cup dairy, 1 ½ tsp. healthy oil

Sweet & Sour Chicken

¼ cup no-salt-added ketchup
¼ cup pineapple juice
3 tbsp. reduced-sodium soy sauce
1 tbsp. rice vinegar
2 tsp. honey
¼ tsp. salt
½ tsp. ground pepper
2 tbsp. toasted sesame oil, divided
1 lb. boneless, skinless chicken breasts, cut into bite-size pieces
8 ounces small broccoli florets
2 cups chopped red bell pepper
1 cup diagonally sliced scallions (1-inch)
3 cups cooked brown rice

Whisk ketchup, pineapple juice, soy sauce, vinegar, honey, salt and pepper in a small bowl. Heat 1 tbsp. oil in a large skillet over high heat. Add chicken and cook, turning occasionally, until browned on all sides, 4 to 5 minutes. Transfer to a plate. Wipe the pan clean; return to high heat and add the remaining 1 tbsp. oil. Add broccoli and bell pepper; cook until charred, about 5 minutes. Add scallions and cook for 1 minute. Return the chicken to the pan and add the ketchup mixture. Cook until bubbly and the sauce coats the chicken. Serve in shallow bowls over rice. Serves 4.Nutritional Information: 465 calories, 5g fat, 1g protein, 38.5 carbohydrate, 66g dietary fiber, 5.9g cholesterol, 6mg sodium.

Nutritional Information: 444 calories; 11.1 g total fat; 63 mg cholesterol; 624 mg sodium. 55.7 g carbohydrates; 29.9 g protein

Live It Tracker: 3 oz.-eq. protein, 2 oz.-eq. grain; 1 cup vegetable

STEPS FOR SPIRITUAL GROWTH

—— GOD'S WORD FOR YOUR LIFE

I have hidden your word in my heart that I might not sin against you.

Psalm 119:11

As you begin to make decisions based on what God's Word teaches you, you will want to memorize what He has promised to those who trust and follow Him. Second Peter 1:3 tells us that God "has given us everything we need for life and godliness through our knowledge of him" (emphasis added). The Bible provides instruction and encouragement for any area of life in which you may be struggling. If you are dealing with a particular emotion or traumatic life event—fear, discouragement, stress, financial upset, the death of a loved one, a relationship difficulty—you can search through a Bible concordance for Scripture passages that deal with that particular situation. Scripture provides great comfort to those who memorize it.

One of the promises of knowing and obeying God's Word is that it gives you wisdom, insight, and understanding above all worldly knowledge (see Psalm 119:97–104). Psalm 119:129–130 says, "Your statutes are wonderful; therefore I obey them. The unfolding of your words gives light; it gives understanding to the simple." Now that's a precious promise about guidance for life!

The Value of Scripture Memory

Scripture memory is an important part of the Christian life. There are four key reasons to memorize Scripture:

1. **TO HANDLE DIFFICULT SITUATIONS.** A heartfelt knowledge of God's Word will equip you to handle any situation that you might face. Declaring such truth as, "I can do everything through Christ" (see Philippians 4:13) and "he will never leave me or forsake me" (see Hebrews 13:5) will enable you to walk through situations with peace and courage.

2. **TO OVERCOME TEMPTATION.** Luke 4:1–13 describes how Jesus used Scripture to overcome His temptations in the desert (see also Matthew 4:1-11). Knowledge of Scripture and the strength that comes with the ability to use it are important parts of putting on the full armor of God in preparation for spiritual warfare (see Ephesians 6:10–18).

3. **TO GET GUIDANCE.** Psalm 119:105 states the Word of God "is a lamp to my feet and a light for my path." You learn to hide God's Word in your heart so His light will direct your decisions and actions throughout your day.

4. **TO TRANSFORM YOUR MIND.** "Do not conform any longer to the pattern of this world, but be transformed by the renewing of your mind" (Romans 12:2). Scripture memory allows you to replace a lie with the truth of God's Word. When Scripture becomes firmly settled in your memory, not only will your thoughts connect with God's thoughts, but you will also be able to honor God with small everyday decisions as well as big life-impacting ones. Scripture memorization is the key to making a permanent lifestyle change in your thought patterns, which brings balance to every other area of your life.

Scripture Memory Tips

- Write the verse down, saying it aloud as you write it.
- Read verses before and after the memory verse to get its context.
- Read the verse several times, emphasizing a different word each time.
- Connect the Scripture reference to the first few words.
- Locate patterns, phrases, or keywords.
- Apply the Scripture to circumstances you are now experiencing.
- Pray the verse, making it personal to your life and inserting your name as the recipient of the promise or teaching. (Try that with 1 Corinthians 10:13, inserting "me" and "I" for "you.")
- Review the verse every day until it becomes second nature to think those words whenever your circumstances match its message. The Holy Spirit will bring the verse to mind when you need it most if you decide to plant it in your memory.

Scripture Memorization Made Easy!

What is your learning style? Do you learn by hearing, by sight, or by doing?

If you learn by hearing—if you are an auditory learner—singing the Scripture memory verses, reading them aloud, or recording them and listening to your recording will be very helpful in the memorization process.

If you are a visual learner, writing the verses and repeatedly reading through them will cement them in your mind.

If you learn by doing—if you are a tactile learner—creating motions for the words or using sign language will enable you to more easily recall the verse.

After determining your learning style, link your Scripture memory with a daily task, such as driving to work, walking on a treadmill, or eating lunch. Use these daily tasks as opportunities to memorize and review your verses.

Meals at home or out with friends can be used as a time to share the verse you are memorizing with those at your table. You could close your personal email messages by typing in your weekly memory verse. Or why not say your memory verse every time you brush your teeth or put on your shoes?

The purpose of Scripture memorization is to be able to apply God's words to your life. If you memorize Scripture using methods that connect with your particular learning style, you will find it easier to hide God's Word in your heart.

—— ESTABLISHING A QUIET TIME

Like all other components of the First Place for Health program, developing a live relationship with God is not a random act. You must intentionally seek God if you are to find Him! It's not that God plays hide-and-seek with you. He is always available to you. He invites you to come boldly into His presence. He reveals Himself to you in the pages of the Bible. And once you decide to earnestly seek Him, you are sure to find Him! When you delight in Him, your gracious God will give you the desires of your heart. Spending time getting to know God involves four basic elements: a priority, a plan, a place, and practice.

A Priority

You can successfully establish a quiet time with God by making this meeting a daily priority. This may require carving out time in your day so you have time and space for this new relationship you are cultivating. Often this will mean eliminating less important things so you will have time and space to meet with God. When speaking about Jesus, John the Baptist said, "He must become greater; I must become less" (John 3:30). You will undoubtedly find that to be true as well. What might you need to eliminate from your current schedule so that spending quality time with God can become a priority?

A Plan

Having made quiet time a priority, you will want to come up with a plan. This plan will include the time you have set aside to spend with God and a general outline of how you will spend your time in God's presence.

Elements you should consider incorporating into your quiet time include:

- Singing a song of praise
- Reading a daily selection in a devotional book or reading a psalm
- Using a systematic Scripture reading plan so you will be exposed to the whole truth of God's Word
- Completing your First Place for Health Bible study for that day
- Praying—silent, spoken, and written prayer
- Writing in your spiritual journal.

You will also want to make a list of the materials you will need to make your encounter with God more meaningful:

- A Bible
- Your First Place for Health Bible study
- Your prayer journal
- A pen and/or pencil
- A devotional book
- A Bible concordance
- A college-level dictionary
- A box of tissues (tears—both of sadness and joy—are often part of our quiet time with God!)

Think of how you would plan an important business meeting or social event, and then transfer that knowledge to your meeting time with God.

A Place

Having formulated a meeting-with-God plan, you will next need to create a meeting-with-God place. Of course, God is always with you; however, in order to have quality devotional time with Him, it is desirable that you find a comfortable meeting place. You will want to select a spot that is quiet and as distraction-free as possible.

Meeting with God in the same place on a regular basis will help you remember what you are there for: to have an encounter with the true and living God!

Having selected the place, put the materials you have determined to use in your quiet time into a basket or on a nearby table or shelf. Now take the time to establish your personal quiet time with God. Tailor your quiet time to fit your needs—and the time you have allotted to spend with God. Although many people elect to meet with God early in the morning, for others afternoon or evening is best. There is no hard-and-fast rule about when your quiet time should be—the only essential thing is that you establish a quiet time!

Start with a small amount of time that you know you can devote yourself to daily. You can be confident that as you consistently spend time with God each day, the amount of time you can spend will increase as you are ready for the next level of your walk with God.

I will meet with God from _____ to _____ daily.

I plan to use that time with God to _____

_____

Supplies I will need to assemble include _____

_____

My meeting place with God will be _____

_____

Practice

After you have chosen the time and place to meet God each day and you have assembled your supplies, there are four easy steps for having a fruitful and worshipful time with the Lord.

STEP 1: Clear Your Heart and Mind

"Be still, and know that I am God" (Psalm 46:10). Begin your quiet time by reading the daily Bible selection from a devotional guide or a psalm. If you are new in your Christian walk, an excellent devotional guide to use is Streams in the Desert by L.B. Cowman. More mature Christians might benefit from My Utmost for His Highest by Oswald Chambers. Of course, you can use any devotional that has a strong emphasis on Scripture and prayer.

STEP 2: Read and Interact with Scripture

"I have hidden your word in my heart that I might not sin against you" (Psalm 119:11). As you open your Bible, ask the Holy Spirit to reveal something He knows you need for this day through the reading of His Word. Always try to find a nugget to encourage or direct you through the day. As you read the passage, pay special attention to the words and phrases the Holy Spirit brings to your attention. Some words may seem to resonate in your soul. You will want to spend time meditating on the passage, asking God what lesson He is teaching you.

After reading the Scripture passage over several times, ask yourself the following questions:

- In light of what I have read today, is there something I must now do? (Confess a sin? Claim a promise? Follow an example? Obey a command? Avoid a situation?)
- How should I respond to what I've read today?

STEP 3: Pray

"Be clear minded and self-controlled so that you can pray" (1 Peter 4:7). Spend time conversing with the Lord in prayer. Prayer is such an important part of First Place for Health that there is an entire section in this member's guide devoted to the practice of prayer.

STEP 4: Praise

"Praise the LORD, O my soul, and forget not all his benefits" (Psalm 103:2). End your quiet time with a time of praise. Be sure to thank the Lord of heaven and warmth for choosing to spend time with you!

—— SHARING YOUR FAITH

Nothing is more effective in drawing someone to Jesus than sharing personal life experiences. People are more open to the good news of Jesus Christ when they see faith in action. Personal faith stories are simple and effective ways to share what Christ is doing in your life, because they show firsthand how Christ makes a difference.

Sharing your faith story has an added benefit: it builds you up in your faith, too! Is your experience in First Place for Health providing you opportunities to share with others what God is doing in your life? If you answered yes, then you have a personal faith story!

If you do not have a personal faith story, perhaps it is because you don't know Jesus Christ as your personal Lord and Savior. Read through "Steps to Becoming a Christian" (which is the next chapter) and begin today to give Christ first place in your life.

Creativity and preparation in using opportunities to share a word or story about Jesus is an important part of the Christian life. Is Jesus helping you in a special way? Are you achieving a level of success or peace that you haven't experienced in other attempts to lose weight, exercise regularly, or eat healthier? As people see you making changes and achieving success, they may ask you how you are doing it. How will—or do—you respond? Remember, your story is unique, and it may allow others to see what Christ is doing in your life. It may also help to bring Christ into the life of another person.

Personal Statements of Faith

First Place for Health gives you a great opportunity to communicate your faith and express what God is doing in your life. Be ready to use your own personal statement of faith whenever the opportunity presents itself. Personal statements of faith should be short and fit naturally into a conversation. They don't require or expect any action or response from the listener. The goal is not to get another person to change but simply to help you communicate who you are and what's important to you.

Here are some examples of short statements of faith that you might use when someone asks what you are doing to lose weight:

- "I've been meeting with a group at my church. We pray together, support each other, learn about nutrition, and study the Bible."

- "It's amazing how Bible study and prayer are helping me lose weight and eat healthier."
- "I've had a lot of support from a group I meet with at church."
- "I'm relying more on God to help me make changes in my lifestyle."

Begin keeping a list of your meaningful experiences as you go through the First Place for Health program. Also notice what is happening in the lives of others. Use the following questions to help you prepare short personal statements and stories of faith:

- What is God doing in your life physically, mentally, emotionally, and spiritually?
- How has your relationship with God changed? Is it more intimate or personal?
- How is prayer, Bible study, and/or the support of others helping you achieve your goals for a healthy weight and good nutrition?

Writing Your Personal Faith Story

Write a brief story about how God is working in your life through First Place for Health. Use your story to help you share with others what's happening in your life.

Use the following questions to help develop your story:

- Why did you join First Place for Health? What specific circumstances led you to a Christ-centered health and weight-loss program? What were you feeling when you joined?
- What was your relationship with Christ when you started First Place for Health? What is it now?
- Has your experience in First Place for Health changed your relationship with Christ? With yourself? With others?
- How has your relationship with Christ, prayer, Bible study, and group support made a difference in your life?
- What specific verse or passage of Scripture has made a difference in the way you view yourself or your relationship with Christ?
- What experiences have impacted your life since starting First Place for Health?
- In what ways is Christ working in your life today? In what ways is He meeting your needs?

- How has Christ worked in other members of your First Place for Health group?

Answer the above questions in a few sentences, and then use your answers to help you write your own short personal faith story.

MEMBER SURVEY

Please answer the following questions to help your leader plan your First Place for Health meeting so that your needs might be met in this session. Give this form to your leader at the first group meeting.

Name _____ Birth date _____

Please list those who live in your household

Name   Relationship   Age
_____
_____
_____
_____

What church do you attend? _____

Would you like to receive more information   Yes   No
about our church?

Occupation _____

What talent or area of expertise would you be willing to share with our class?
_____
_____

Why did you join First Place for Health?
_____
_____

With notice, would you be willing to lead a Bible study   Yes   No
discussion one week?

Are you comfortable praying out loud? _____

If the assistant leader were absent, would you be willing   Yes   No
to assist weighing in memebers and possibly evaluating
the Live It Trackers?

Any other comments:
_____
_____

PERSONAL WEIGHT AND MEASUREMENT RECORD

WEEK	WEIGHT	+ OR -	GOAL THIS SESSION	POUNDS TO GOAL
1				
2				
3				
4				
5				
6				
7				
8				
9				
10				
11				
12				

BEGINNING MEASUREMENTS

WAIST_____ HIPS_____ THIGHS_____ CHEST_____

ENDING MEASUREMENTS

WAIST_____ HIPS_____ THIGHS_____ CHEST_____

It is for freedom that Christ has set us free. Stand firm, then, and do not let yourselves be burdened again by a yoke of slavery..

GALATIANS 5:1

Date: _____

Name: _____

Home   Phone: _____

Work   Phone: _____

Email: _____

Personal Prayer Concernts

_____

_____

_____

_____

_____

_____

_____

_____

This form is for prayer requests that are personal to you and your journey in First Place for Health. Please complete and have it ready to turn in when you arrive at your group meeting.

The Lord will fight for you while you keep silent.
EXODUS 14:14

Date: _____

Name: _____

Home   Phone: _____

Work   Phone: _____

Email: _____

Personal Prayer Concernts

_____

_____

_____

_____

_____

_____

_____

_____

This form is for prayer requests that are personal to you and your journey in First Place for Health. Please complete and have it ready to turn in when you arrive at your group meeting.

From now on let no one cause me trouble, for I bear on my body the
marks of Jesus.

GALATIANS 6: 17

Date: _____

Name: _____

Home   Phone: _____

Work   Phone: _____

Email: _____

Personal Prayer Concernts

_____

_____

_____

_____

_____

_____

_____

_____

This form is for prayer requests that are personal to you and your journey in First Place for Health. Please complete and have it ready to turn in when you arrive at your group meeting.

"See, the former things have taken place, and new things I declare;
before they spring into being I announce them to you."

ISAIAH 42: 9

Date: _____

Name: _____

Home Phone: _____

Work Phone: _____

Email: _____

Personal Prayer Concernts

_____

_____

_____

_____

_____

_____

_____

This form is for prayer requests that are personal to you and your journey in First Place for Health. Please complete and have it ready to turn in when you arrive at your group meeting.

But the seed falling on good soil refers to someone who hears the word
and understands it.

MATTHEW 13:23

Date: _____

Name: _____

Home   Phone: _____

Work   Phone: _____

Email: _____

Personal Prayer Concernts

_____

_____

_____

_____

_____

_____

_____

This form is for prayer requests that are personal to you and your journey in First Place for Health. Please complete and have it ready to turn in when you arrive at your group meeting.

He told them, "The harvest is plentiful, but the workers are few. Ask the
Lord of the harvest, therefore, to send out workers into his harvest field."

LUKE 10: 2

Date: _____

Name: _____

Home   Phone: _____

Work   Phone: _____

Email: _____

Personal Prayer Concernts

_____

_____

_____

_____

_____

_____

_____

This form is for prayer requests that are personal to you and your journey in First Place for Health.
Please complete and have it ready to turn in when you arrive at your group meeting.

PRAYER PARTNER

Devote yourselves to prayer, being watchful and thankful.

COLOSSIANS 4:2

Date: _____

Name: _____

Home   Phone: _____

Work   Phone: _____

Email: _____

Personal Prayer Concernts

_____

_____

_____

_____

_____

_____

_____

_____

This form is for prayer requests that are personal to you and your journey in First Place for Health. Please complete and have it ready to turn in when you arrive at your group meeting.

Do you not know that in a race all the runners run, but only one gets the
prize? Run in such a way to get the prize.

1 CORINTHIANS 9:24

Date: _____

Name: _____

Home   Phone: _____

Work   Phone: _____

Email: _____

Personal Prayer Concernts

_____

_____

_____

_____

_____

_____

_____

This form is for prayer requests that are personal to you and your journey in First Place for Health.
Please complete and have it ready to turn in when you arrive at your group meeting.

No discipline seems pleasant at the time, but painful. Later on, however, it produces a harvest of righteousness and peace for those who have been trained by it.

HEBREWS 12:11

Date: _____

Name: _____

Home   Phone: _____

Work   Phone: _____

Email: _____

Personal Prayer Concernts

_____

_____

_____

_____

_____

_____

_____

_____

May he give you the desire of your heart and make all your plans suc-

ceed.

PSALM 20:4

Date: _____

Name: _____

Home   Phone: _____

Work   Phone: _____

Email: _____

Personal Prayer Concernts

_____

_____

_____

_____

_____

_____

_____

_____

This form is for prayer requests that are personal to you and your journey in First Place for Health. Please complete and have it ready to turn in when you arrive at your group meeting.

Date: _____

Name: _____

Home Phone: _____

Work Phone: _____

Email: _____

Personal Prayer Concernts

_____

_____

_____

_____

_____

_____

_____

This form is for prayer requests that are personal to you and your journey in First Place for Health. Please complete and have it ready to turn in when you arrive at your group meeting.

100-MILE CLUB

WALKING			
slowly, 2 mph	30 min =	156 cal =	1 mile
moderately, 3 mph	20 min =	156 cal =	1 mile
very briskly, 4 mph	15 min =	156 cal =	1 mile
speed walking	10 min =	156 cal =	1 mile
up stairs	13 min =	159 cal =	1 mile
RUNNING / JOGGING			
. . .	10 min =	156 cal =	1 mile
CYCLE OUTDOORS			
slowly, < 10 mph	20 min =	156 cal =	1 mile
light effort, 10-12 mph	12 min =	156 cal =	1 mile
moderate effort, 12-14 mph	10 min =	156 cal =	1 mile
vigorous effort, 14-16 mph	7.5 min =	156 cal =	1 mile
very fast, 16-19 mph	6.5 min =	152 cal =	1 mile
SPORTS ACTIVITIES			
playing tennis (singles)	10 min =	156 cal =	1 mile
swimming			
light to moderate effort	11 min =	152 cal =	1 mile
fast, vigorous effort	7.5 min =	156 cal =	1 mile
softball	15 min =	156 cal =	1 mile
golf	20 min =	156 cal =	1 mile
rollerblading	6.5 min =	152 cal =	1 mile
ice skating	11 min =	152 cal =	1 mile
jumping rope	7.5 min =	156 cal =	1 mile
basketball	12 min =	156 cal =	1 mile
soccer (casual)	15 min =	159 min =	1 mile
AROUND THE HOUSE			
mowing grass	22 min =	156 cal =	1 mile
mopping, sweeping, vacuuming	19.5 min =	155 cal =	1 mile
cooking	40 min =	160 cal =	1 mile
gardening	19 min =	156 cal =	1 mile
housework (general)	35 min =	156 cal =	1 mile

AROUND THE HOUSE			
ironing	45 min =	153 cal =	1 mile
raking leaves	25 min =	150 cal =	1 mile
washing car	23 min =	156 cal =	1 mile
washing dishes	45 min =	153 cal =	1 mile
AT THE GYM			
stair machine	8.5 min =	155 cal =	1 mile
stationary bike			
slowly, 10 mph	30 min =	156 cal =	1 mile
moderately, 10-13 mph	15 min =	156 cal =	1 mile
vigorously, 13-16 mph	7.5 min =	156 cal =	1 mile
briskly, 16-19 mph	6.5 min =	156 cal =	1 mile
elliptical trainer	12 min =	156 cal =	1 mile
weight machines (vigorously)	13 min =	152 cal =	1 mile
aerobics			
low impact	15 min =	156 cal =	1 mile
high impact	12 min =	156 cal =	1 mile
water	20 min =	156 cal =	1 mile
pilates	15 min =	156 cal =	1 mile
raquetball (casual)	15 min =	156 cal =	1 mile
stretching exercises	25 min =	150 cal =	1 mile
weight lifting (also works for weight machines used moderately or gently)	30 min =	156 cal =	1 mile
FAMILY LEISURE			
playing piano	37 min =	155 cal =	1 mile
jumping rope	10 min =	152 cal =	1 mile
skating (moderate)	20 min =	152 cal =	1 mile
swimming			
moderate	17 min =	156 cal =	1 mile
vigorous	10 min =	148 cal =	1 mile
table tennis	25 min =	150 cal =	1 mile
walk / run / play with kids	25 min =	150 cal =	1 mile

LIVE IT TRACKER

Name: _____

My activity goal for next week:
○ None   ○ <30 min/day   ○ 30-60 min/day

My food goal for next week: _____
_____

Date: _____ Week #: _____

loss / gain _____ Calorie Range: _____

My week at a glance:
○ Great   ○ So-so   ○ Not so great

Activity level:
○ None   ○ <30 min/day   ○ 30-60 min/day

RECOMMENDED DAILY AMOUNT OF FOOD FROM EACH GROUP

GROUP	DAILY CALORIES							
	1300-1400	1500-1600	1700-1800	1900-2000	2100-2200	2300-2400	2500-2600	2700-2800
Fruits	1.5 – 2 c.	1.5 – 2 c.	1.5 – 2 c.	2 – 2.5 c.	2 – 2.5 c.	2.5 – 3.5 c.	3.5 – 4.5 c.	3.5 – 4.5 c.
Vegetables	1.5 – 2 c.	2 – 2.5 c.	2.5 – 3 c.	2.5 – 3 c.	3 – 3.5 c.	3.5 – 4.5 c..	4.5 – 5 c.	4.5 – 5 c.
Grains	5 oz eq.	5-6 oz eq.	6-7 oz eq.	6-7 oz eq.	7-8 oz eq.	8-9 oz eq.	9-10 oz eq.	10-11 oz eq.
Dairy	2-3 c.	3 c.	3 c.	3 c.	3 c.	3 c.	3 c.	3 c.
Protein	4 oz eq.	5 oz eq.	5-5.5 oz eq.	5.5-6.5 oz eq.	6.5-7 oz eq.	7-7.5 oz eq.	7-7.5 oz eq.	7.5-8 oz eq.
Healthy Oils & Other Fats	4 tsp.	5 tsp.	5 tsp.	6 tsp.	6 tsp.	7 tsp.	8 tsp.	8 tsp.
Water & Super Beverages*	Women: 9 c. Men: 13 c.	Women: 9 c. Men: 13 c.	Women: 9 c. Men: 13 c.	Women: 9 c. Men: 13 c.	Women: 9 c. Men: 13 c.	Women: 9 c. Men: 13 c.	Women: 9 c. Men: 13 c.	Women: 9 c. Men: 13 c.

*May count up to 3 cups caffeinated tea or coffee toward goal

DAILY FOOD GROUP TRACKER

GROUP	FRUITS	VEGETABLES	GRAINS	PROTEIN	DAIRY	HEALTHY OILS & OTHER FATS	WATER & SUPER BEVERAGES
❶ Estimate Total							
❷ Estimate Total							
❸ Estimate Total							
❹ Estimate Total							
❺ Estimate Total							
❻ Estimate Total							
❼ Estimate Total							

FOOD CHOICES   DAY ❶

Breakfast: _____
Lunch: _____
Dinner: _____
Snacks: _____

PHYSICAL ACTIVITY   steps/miles/minutes: _____

description: _____
_____

SPIRITUAL ACTIVITY

description: _____
_____

FOOD CHOICES DAY ❷

Breakfast: _____
Lunch: _____
Dinner: _____
Snacks: _____

PHYSICAL ACTIVITY   steps/miles/minutes: _____

description: _____

SPIRITUAL ACTIVITY

description: _____

FOOD CHOICES DAY ❸

Breakfast: _____
Lunch: _____
Dinner: _____
Snacks: _____

PHYSICAL ACTIVITY   steps/miles/minutes: _____

description: _____

SPIRITUAL ACTIVITY

description: _____

FOOD CHOICES DAY ❹

Breakfast: _____
Lunch: _____
Dinner: _____
Snacks: _____

PHYSICAL ACTIVITY   steps/miles/minutes: _____

description: _____

SPIRITUAL ACTIVITY

description: _____

FOOD CHOICES DAY ❺

Breakfast: _____
Lunch: _____
Dinner: _____
Snacks: _____

PHYSICAL ACTIVITY   steps/miles/minutes: _____

description: _____

SPIRITUAL ACTIVITY

description: _____

FOOD CHOICES DAY ❻

Breakfast: _____
Lunch: _____
Dinner: _____
Snacks: _____

PHYSICAL ACTIVITY   steps/miles/minutes: _____

description: _____

SPIRITUAL ACTIVITY

description: _____

FOOD CHOICES DAY ❼

Breakfast: _____
Lunch: _____
Dinner: _____
Snacks: _____

PHYSICAL ACTIVITY   steps/miles/minutes: _____

description: _____

SPIRITUAL ACTIVITY

description: _____

LIVE IT TRACKER

Name: _____

Date: _____ Week #: _____

My activity goal for next week:
○ None   ○ <30 min/day   ○ 30-60 min/day

loss/gain _____   Calorie Range: _____

My week at a glance:
○ Great   ○ So-so   ○ Not so great

My food goal for next week: _____

Activity level:
○ None   ○ <30 min/day   ○ 30-60 min/day

RECOMMENDED DAILY AMOUNT OF FOOD FROM EACH GROUP

GROUP	DAILY CALORIES							
....	1300-1400	1500-1600	1700-1800	1900-2000	2100-2200	2300-2400	2500-2600	2700-2800
Fruits	1.5 – 2 c.	1.5 – 2 c.	1.5 – 2 c.	2 – 2.5 c.	2 – 2.5 c.	2.5 – 3.5 c.	3.5 – 4.5 c.	3.5 – 4.5 c.
Vegetables	1.5 – 2 c.	2 – 2.5 c.	2.5 – 3 c.	2.5 – 3 c.	3 – 3.5 c.	3.5 – 4.5 c..	4.5 – 5 c.	4.5 – 5 c.
Grains	5 oz eq.	5-6 oz eq.	6-7 oz eq.	6-7 oz eq.	7-8 oz eq.	8-9 oz eq.	9-10 oz eq.	10-11 oz eq.
Dairy	2-3 c.	3 c.	3 c.	3 c.	3 c.	3 c.	3 c.	3 c.
Protein	4 oz eq.	5 oz eq.	5-5.5 oz eq.	5.5-6.5 oz eq.	6.5-7 oz eq.	7-7.5 oz eq.	7-7.5 oz eq.	7.5-8 oz eq.
Healthy Oils & Other Fats	4 tsp.	5 tsp.	5 tsp.	6 tsp.	6 tsp.	7 tsp.	8 tsp.	8 tsp.
Water & Super Beverages*	Women: 9 c. Men: 13 c.	Women: 9 c. Men: 13 c.	Women: 9 c. Men: 13 c.	Women: 9 c. Men: 13 c.	Women: 9 c. Men: 13 c.	Women: 9 c. Men: 13 c.	Women: 9 c. Men: 13 c.	Women: 9 c. Men: 13 c.

*May count up to 3 cups caffeinated tea or coffee toward goal

DAILY FOOD GROUP TRACKER

GROUP	FRUITS	VEGETABLES	GRAINS	PROTEIN	DAIRY	HEALTHY OILS & OTHER FATS	WATER & SUPER BEVERAGES
1 Estimate Total							
2 Estimate Total							
3 Estimate Total							
4 Estimate Total							
5 Estimate Total							
6 Estimate Total							
7 Estimate Total							

FOOD CHOICES   DAY ❶

Breakfast: _____

Lunch: _____

Dinner: _____

Snacks: _____

PHYSICAL ACTIVITY   steps/miles/minutes: _____

description: _____

SPIRITUAL ACTIVITY

description: _____

FOOD CHOICES   DAY **2**

Breakfast: _____

Lunch: _____

Dinner: _____

Snacks: _____

PHYSICAL ACTIVITY steps/miles/minutes:_____ | **SPIRITUAL ACTIVITY**

description: _____ | description: _____

FOOD CHOICES   DAY **3**

Breakfast: _____

Lunch: _____

Dinner: _____

Snacks: _____

PHYSICAL ACTIVITY steps/miles/minutes:_____ | **SPIRITUAL ACTIVITY**

description: _____ | description: _____

FOOD CHOICES   DAY **4**

Breakfast: _____

Lunch: _____

Dinner: _____

Snacks: _____

PHYSICAL ACTIVITY steps/miles/minutes:_____ | **SPIRITUAL ACTIVITY**

description: _____ | description: _____

FOOD CHOICES   DAY **5**

Breakfast: _____

Lunch: _____

Dinner: _____

Snacks: _____

PHYSICAL ACTIVITY steps/miles/minutes:_____ | **SPIRITUAL ACTIVITY**

description: _____ | description: _____

FOOD CHOICES   DAY **6**

Breakfast: _____

Lunch: _____

Dinner: _____

Snacks: _____

PHYSICAL ACTIVITY steps/miles/minutes:_____ | **SPIRITUAL ACTIVITY**

description: _____ | description: _____

FOOD CHOICES   DAY **7**

Breakfast: _____

Lunch: _____

Dinner: _____

Snacks: _____

PHYSICAL ACTIVITY steps/miles/minutes:_____ | **SPIRITUAL ACTIVITY**

description: _____ | description: _____

LIVE IT TRACKER

Name: _____

Date: _____ Week #: _____

My activity goal for next week:
○ None   ○ <30 min/day   ○ 30-60 min/day

loss/gain _____ Calorie Range: _____

My food goal for next week: _____
_____

My week at a glance:
○ Great   ○ So-so   ○ Not so great

Activity level:
○ None   ○ <30 min/day   ○ 30-60 min/day

RECOMMENDED DAILY AMOUNT OF FOOD FROM EACH GROUP

GROUP	DAILY CALORIES							
....	1300-1400	1500-1600	1700-1800	1900-2000	2100-2200	2300-2400	2500-2600	2700-2800
Fruits	1.5 – 2 c.	1.5 – 2 c.	1.5 – 2 c.	2 – 2.5 c.	2 – 2.5 c.	2.5 – 3.5 c.	3.5 – 4.5 c.	3.5 – 4.5 c.
Vegetables	1.5 – 2 c.	2 – 2.5 c.	2.5 – 3 c.	2.5 – 3 c.	3 – 3.5 c.	3.5 – 4.5 c..	4.5 – 5 c.	4.5 – 5 c.
Grains	5 oz eq.	5-6 oz eq.	6-7 oz eq.	6-7 oz eq.	7-8 oz eq.	8-9 oz eq.	9-10 oz eq.	10-11 oz eq.
Dairy	2-3 c.	3 c.	3 c.	3 c.	3 c.	3 c.	3 c.	3 c.
Protein	4 oz eq.	5 oz eq.	5-5.5 oz eq.	5.5-6.5 oz eq.	6.5-7 oz eq.	7-7.5 oz eq.	7-7.5 oz eq.	7.5-8 oz eq.
Healthy Oils & Other Fats	4 tsp.	5 tsp.	5 tsp.	6 tsp.	6 tsp.	7 tsp.	8 tsp.	8 tsp.
Water & Super Beverages*	Women: 9 c. Men: 13 c.	Women: 9 c. Men: 13 c.	Women: 9 c. Men: 13 c.	Women: 9 c. Men: 13 c.	Women: 9 c. Men: 13 c.	Women: 9 c. Men: 13 c.	Women: 9 c. Men: 13 c.	Women: 9 c. Men: 13 c.

*May count up to 3 cups caffeinated tea or coffee toward goal

DAILY FOOD GROUP TRACKER

GROUP	FRUITS	VEGETABLES	GRAINS	PROTEIN	DAIRY	HEALTHY OILS & OTHER FATS	WATER & SUPER BEVERAGES
① Estimate Total							
② Estimate Total							
③ Estimate Total							
④ Estimate Total							
⑤ Estimate Total							
⑥ Estimate Total							
⑦ Estimate Total							

FOOD CHOICES   DAY ❶

Breakfast: _____
Lunch: _____
Dinner: _____
Snacks: _____

PHYSICAL ACTIVITY   steps/miles/minutes: _____

description: _____
_____

SPIRITUAL ACTIVITY

description: _____
_____

FOOD CHOICES   DAY ❷

Breakfast: _____
Lunch: _____
Dinner: _____
Snacks: _____

PHYSICAL ACTIVITY   steps/miles/minutes:_____   **SPIRITUAL ACTIVITY**

description: _____   description: _____

FOOD CHOICES   DAY ❸

Breakfast: _____
Lunch: _____
Dinner: _____
Snacks: _____

PHYSICAL ACTIVITY   steps/miles/minutes:_____   **SPIRITUAL ACTIVITY**

description: _____   description: _____

FOOD CHOICES   DAY ❹

Breakfast: _____
Lunch: _____
Dinner: _____
Snacks: _____

PHYSICAL ACTIVITY   steps/miles/minutes:_____   **SPIRITUAL ACTIVITY**

description: _____   description: _____

FOOD CHOICES   DAY ❺

Breakfast: _____
Lunch: _____
Dinner: _____
Snacks: _____

PHYSICAL ACTIVITY   steps/miles/minutes:_____   **SPIRITUAL ACTIVITY**

description: _____   description: _____

FOOD CHOICES   DAY ❻

Breakfast: _____
Lunch: _____
Dinner: _____
Snacks: _____

PHYSICAL ACTIVITY   steps/miles/minutes:_____   **SPIRITUAL ACTIVITY**

description: _____   description: _____

FOOD CHOICES   DAY ❼

Breakfast: _____
Lunch: _____
Dinner: _____
Snacks: _____

PHYSICAL ACTIVITY   steps/miles/minutes:_____   **SPIRITUAL ACTIVITY**

description: _____   description: _____

LIVE IT TRACKER

Name: _____

Date: _____ Week #: _____

My activity goal for next week:
○ None   ○ <30 min/day   ○ 30-60 min/day

My food goal for next week: _____
_____

loss/gain _____ Calorie Range: _____

My week at a glance:
○ Great   ○ So-so   ○ Not so great

Activity level:
○ None   ○ <30 min/day   ○ 30-60 min/day

RECOMMENDED DAILY AMOUNT OF FOOD FROM EACH GROUP

GROUP	DAILY CALORIES							
	1300-1400	1500-1600	1700-1800	1900-2000	2100-2200	2300-2400	2500-2600	2700-2800
Fruits	1.5 – 2 c.	1.5 – 2 c.	1.5 – 2 c.	2 – 2.5 c.	2 – 2.5 c.	2.5 – 3.5 c.	3.5 – 4.5 c.	3.5 – 4.5 c.
Vegetables	1.5 – 2 c.	2 – 2.5 c.	2.5 – 3 c.	2.5 – 3 c.	3 – 3.5 c.	3.5 – 4.5 c..	4.5 – 5 c.	4.5 – 5 c.
Grains	5 oz eq.	5-6 oz eq.	6-7 oz eq.	6-7 oz eq.	7-8 oz eq.	8-9 oz eq.	9-10 oz eq.	10-11 oz eq.
Dairy	2-3 c.	3 c.	3 c.	3 c.	3 c.	3 c.	3 c.	3 c.
Protein	4 oz eq.	5 oz eq.	5-5.5 oz eq.	5.5-6.5 oz eq.	6.5-7 oz eq.	7-7.5 oz eq.	7-7.5 oz eq.	7.5-8 oz eq.
Healthy Oils & Other Fats	4 tsp.	5 tsp.	5 tsp.	6 tsp.	6 tsp.	7 tsp.	8 tsp.	8 tsp.
Water & Super Beverages*	Women: 9 c. Men: 13 c.	Women: 9 c. Men: 13 c.	Women: 9 c. Men: 13 c.	Women: 9 c. Men: 13 c.	Women: 9 c. Men: 13 c.	Women: 9 c. Men: 13 c.	Women: 9 c. Men: 13 c.	Women: 9 c. Men: 13 c.

*May count up to 3 cups caffeinated tea or coffee toward goal

DAILY FOOD GROUP TRACKER

GROUP	FRUITS	VEGETABLES	GRAINS	PROTEIN	DAIRY	HEALTHY OILS & OTHER FATS	WATER & SUPER BEVERAGES
① Estimate Total							
② Estimate Total							
③ Estimate Total							
④ Estimate Total							
⑤ Estimate Total							
⑥ Estimate Total							
⑦ Estimate Total							

FOOD CHOICES   DAY ❶

Breakfast: _____
Lunch: _____
Dinner: _____
Snacks: _____

PHYSICAL ACTIVITY   steps/miles/minutes: _____

description: _____
_____

SPIRITUAL ACTIVITY

description: _____
_____

FOOD CHOICES   DAY ❷

Breakfast: _____

Lunch: _____

Dinner: _____

Snacks: _____

PHYSICAL ACTIVITY   steps/miles/minutes:_____ | ### SPIRITUAL ACTIVITY

description: _____ | description: _____

FOOD CHOICES   DAY ❸

Breakfast: _____

Lunch: _____

Dinner: _____

Snacks: _____

PHYSICAL ACTIVITY   steps/miles/minutes:_____ | ### SPIRITUAL ACTIVITY

description: _____ | description: _____

FOOD CHOICES   DAY ❹

Breakfast: _____

Lunch: _____

Dinner: _____

Snacks: _____

PHYSICAL ACTIVITY   steps/miles/minutes:_____ | ### SPIRITUAL ACTIVITY

description: _____ | description: _____

FOOD CHOICES   DAY ❺

Breakfast: _____

Lunch: _____

Dinner: _____

Snacks: _____

PHYSICAL ACTIVITY   steps/miles/minutes:_____ | ### SPIRITUAL ACTIVITY

description: _____ | description: _____

FOOD CHOICES   DAY ❻

Breakfast: _____

Lunch: _____

Dinner: _____

Snacks: _____

PHYSICAL ACTIVITY   steps/miles/minutes:_____ | ### SPIRITUAL ACTIVITY

description: _____ | description: _____

FOOD CHOICES   DAY ❼

Breakfast: _____

Lunch: _____

Dinner: _____

Snacks: _____

PHYSICAL ACTIVITY   steps/miles/minutes:_____ | ### SPIRITUAL ACTIVITY

description: _____ | description: _____

LIVE IT TRACKER

Name: _____

Date: _____ Week #: _____

My activity goal for next week:
○ None   ○ <30 min/day   ○ 30-60 min/day

loss / gain _____ Calorie Range: _____

My food goal for next week: _____
_____

My week at a glance:
○ Great   ○ So-so   ○ Not so great

Activity level:
○ None   ○ <30 min/day   ○ 30-60 min/day

RECOMMENDED DAILY AMOUNT OF FOOD FROM EACH GROUP

GROUP	DAILY CALORIES							
....	1300-1400	1500-1600	1700-1800	1900-2000	2100-2200	2300-2400	2500-2600	2700-2800
Fruits	1.5 – 2 c.	1.5 – 2 c.	1.5 – 2 c.	2 – 2.5 c.	2 – 2.5 c.	2.5 – 3.5 c.	3.5 – 4.5 c.	3.5 – 4.5 c.
Vegetables	1.5 – 2 c.	2 – 2.5 c.	2.5 – 3 c.	2.5 – 3 c.	3 – 3.5 c.	3.5 – 4.5 c..	4.5 – 5 c.	4.5 – 5 c.
Grains	5 oz eq.	5-6 oz eq.	6-7 oz eq.	6-7 oz eq.	7-8 oz eq.	8-9 oz eq.	9-10 oz eq.	10-11 oz eq.
Dairy	2-3 c.	3 c.	3 c.	3 c.	3 c.	3 c.	3 c.	3 c.
Protein	4 oz eq.	5 oz eq.	5-5.5 oz eq.	5.5-6.5 oz eq.	6.5-7 oz eq.	7-7.5 oz eq.	7-7.5 oz eq.	7.5-8 oz eq.
Healthy Oils & Other Fats	4 tsp.	5 tsp.	5 tsp.	6 tsp.	6 tsp.	7 tsp.	8 tsp.	8 tsp.
Water & Super Beverages*	Women: 9 c. Men: 13 c.	Women: 9 c. Men: 13 c.	Women: 9 c. Men: 13 c.	Women: 9 c. Men: 13 c.	Women: 9 c. Men: 13 c.	Women: 9 c. Men: 13 c.	Women: 9 c. Men: 13 c.	Women: 9 c. Men: 13 c.

*May count up to 3 cups caffeinated tea or coffee toward goal

DAILY FOOD GROUP TRACKER

GROUP	FRUITS	VEGETABLES	GRAINS	PROTEIN	DAIRY	HEALTHY OILS & OTHER FATS	WATER & SUPER BEVERAGES
① Estimate Total							
② Estimate Total							
③ Estimate Total							
④ Estimate Total							
⑤ Estimate Total							
⑥ Estimate Total							
⑦ Estimate Total							

FOOD CHOICES   DAY ❶

Breakfast: _____
Lunch: _____
Dinner: _____
Snacks: _____

PHYSICAL ACTIVITY   steps/miles/minutes: _____

description: _____
_____

SPIRITUAL ACTIVITY

description: _____
_____

FOOD CHOICES

DAY 2

Breakfast: _____

Lunch: _____

Dinner: _____

Snacks: _____

PHYSICAL ACTIVITY   steps/miles/minutes: _____   **SPIRITUAL ACTIVITY**

description: _____   description: _____

FOOD CHOICES

DAY 3

Breakfast: _____

Lunch: _____

Dinner: _____

Snacks: _____

PHYSICAL ACTIVITY   steps/miles/minutes: _____   **SPIRITUAL ACTIVITY**

description: _____   description: _____

FOOD CHOICES

DAY 4

Breakfast: _____

Lunch: _____

Dinner: _____

Snacks: _____

PHYSICAL ACTIVITY   steps/miles/minutes: _____   **SPIRITUAL ACTIVITY**

description: _____   description: _____

FOOD CHOICES

DAY 5

Breakfast: _____

Lunch: _____

Dinner: _____

Snacks: _____

PHYSICAL ACTIVITY   steps/miles/minutes: _____   **SPIRITUAL ACTIVITY**

description: _____   description: _____

FOOD CHOICES

DAY 6

Breakfast: _____

Lunch: _____

Dinner: _____

Snacks: _____

PHYSICAL ACTIVITY   steps/miles/minutes: _____   **SPIRITUAL ACTIVITY**

description: _____   description: _____

FOOD CHOICES

DAY 7

Breakfast: _____

Lunch: _____

Dinner: _____

Snacks: _____

PHYSICAL ACTIVITY   steps/miles/minutes: _____   **SPIRITUAL ACTIVITY**

description: _____   description: _____

Name: _____

My activity goal for next week:
○ None   ○ <30 min/day   ○ 30-60 min/day

My food goal for next week: _____

Date: _____ Week #: _____

loss / gain _____ Calorie Range: _____

My week at a glance:
○ Great   ○ So-so   ○ Not so great

Activity level:
○ None   ○ <30 min/day   ○ 30-60 min/day

RECOMMENDED DAILY AMOUNT OF FOOD FROM EACH GROUP

GROUP ·······	DAILY CALORIES							
	1300-1400	1500-1600	1700-1800	1900-2000	2100-2200	2300-2400	2500-2600	2700-2800
Fruits	1.5 – 2 c.	1.5 – 2 c.	1.5 – 2 c.	2 – 2.5 c.	2 – 2.5 c.	2.5 – 3.5 c.	3.5 – 4.5 c.	3.5 – 4.5 c.
Vegetables	1.5 – 2 c.	2 – 2.5 c.	2.5 – 3 c.	2.5 – 3 c.	3 – 3.5 c.	3.5 – 4.5 c..	4.5 – 5 c.	4.5 – 5 c.
Grains	5 oz eq.	5-6 oz eq.	6-7 oz eq.	6-7 oz eq.	7-8 oz eq.	8-9 oz eq.	9-10 oz eq.	10-11 oz eq.
Dairy	2-3 c.	3 c.	3 c.	3 c.	3 c.	3 c.	3 c.	3 c.
Protein	4 oz eq.	5 oz eq.	5-5.5 oz eq.	5.5-6.5 oz eq.	6.5-7 oz eq.	7-7.5 oz eq.	7-7.5 oz eq.	7.5-8 oz eq.
Healthy Oils & Other Fats	4 tsp.	5 tsp.	5 tsp.	6 tsp.	6 tsp.	7 tsp.	8 tsp.	8 tsp.
Water & Super Beverages*	Women: 9 c. Men: 13 c.	Women: 9 c. Men: 13 c.	Women: 9 c. Men: 13 c.	Women: 9 c. Men: 13 c.	Women: 9 c. Men: 13 c.	Women: 9 c. Men: 13 c.	Women: 9 c. Men: 13 c.	Women: 9 c. Men: 13 c.

*May count up to 3 cups caffeinated tea or coffee toward goal

DAILY FOOD GROUP TRACKER

GROUP	FRUITS	VEGETABLES	GRAINS	PROTEIN	DAIRY	HEALTHY OILS & OTHER FATS	WATER & SUPER BEVERAGES
❶ Estimate Total							
❷ Estimate Total							
❸ Estimate Total							
❹ Estimate Total							
❺ Estimate Total							
❻ Estimate Total							
❼ Estimate Total							

FOOD CHOICES **DAY ❶**

Breakfast: _____

Lunch: _____

Dinner: _____

Snacks: _____

PHYSICAL ACTIVITY   steps/miles/minutes: _____

description: _____

SPIRITUAL ACTIVITY

description: _____

FOOD CHOICES   DAY ❷

Breakfast: _____

Lunch: _____

Dinner: _____

Snacks: _____

PHYSICAL ACTIVITY   steps/miles/minutes:_____   **SPIRITUAL ACTIVITY**

description: _____   description: _____

FOOD CHOICES   DAY ❸

Breakfast: _____

Lunch: _____

Dinner: _____

Snacks: _____

PHYSICAL ACTIVITY   steps/miles/minutes:_____   **SPIRITUAL ACTIVITY**

description: _____   description: _____

FOOD CHOICES   DAY ❹

Breakfast: _____

Lunch: _____

Dinner: _____

Snacks: _____

PHYSICAL ACTIVITY   steps/miles/minutes:_____   **SPIRITUAL ACTIVITY**

description: _____   description: _____

FOOD CHOICES   DAY ❺

Breakfast: _____

Lunch: _____

Dinner: _____

Snacks: _____

PHYSICAL ACTIVITY   steps/miles/minutes:_____   **SPIRITUAL ACTIVITY**

description: _____   description: _____

FOOD CHOICES   DAY ❻

Breakfast: _____

Lunch: _____

Dinner: _____

Snacks: _____

PHYSICAL ACTIVITY   steps/miles/minutes:_____   **SPIRITUAL ACTIVITY**

description: _____   description: _____

FOOD CHOICES   DAY ❼

Breakfast: _____

Lunch: _____

Dinner: _____

Snacks: _____

PHYSICAL ACTIVITY   steps/miles/minutes:_____   **SPIRITUAL ACTIVITY**

description: _____   description: _____

LIVE IT TRACKER

Name: _____

Date: _____ Week #: _____

My activity goal for next week:
○ None ○ <30 min/day ○ 30-60 min/day

loss / gain _____ Calorie Range: _____

My food goal for next week: _____

My week at a glance:
○ Great ○ So-so ○ Not so great

Activity level:
○ None ○ <30 min/day ○ 30-60 min/day

RECOMMENDED DAILY AMOUNT OF FOOD FROM EACH GROUP

DAILY CALORIES

GROUP	1300-1400	1500-1600	1700-1800	1900-2000	2100-2200	2300-2400	2500-2600	2700-2800
Fruits	1.5 – 2 c.	1.5 – 2 c.	1.5 – 2 c.	2 – 2.5 c.	2 – 2.5 c.	2.5 – 3.5 c.	3.5 – 4.5 c.	3.5 – 4.5 c.
Vegetables	1.5 – 2 c.	2 – 2.5 c.	2.5 – 3 c.	2.5 – 3 c.	3 – 3.5 c.	3.5 – 4.5 c..	4.5 – 5 c.	4.5 – 5 c.
Grains	5 oz eq.	5-6 oz eq.	6-7 oz eq.	6-7 oz eq.	7-8 oz eq.	8-9 oz eq.	9-10 oz eq.	10-11 oz eq.
Dairy	2-3 c.	3 c.	3 c.	3 c.	3 c.	3 c.	3 c.	3 c.
Protein	4 oz eq.	5 oz eq.	5-5.5 oz eq.	5.5-6.5 oz eq.	6.5-7 oz eq.	7-7.5 oz eq.	7-7.5 oz eq.	7.5-8 oz eq.
Healthy Oils & Other Fats	4 tsp.	5 tsp.	5 tsp.	6 tsp.	6 tsp.	7 tsp.	8 tsp.	8 tsp.
Water & Super Beverages*	Women: 9 c. Men: 13 c.	Women: 9 c. Men: 13 c.	Women: 9 c. Men: 13 c.	Women: 9 c. Men: 13 c.	Women: 9 c. Men: 13 c.	Women: 9 c. Men: 13 c.	Women: 9 c. Men: 13 c.	Women: 9 c. Men: 13 c.

*May count up to 3 cups caffeinated tea or coffee toward goal

DAILY FOOD GROUP TRACKER

GROUP	FRUITS	VEGETABLES	GRAINS	PROTEIN	DAIRY	HEALTHY OILS & OTHER FATS	WATER & SUPER BEVERAGES
1 Estimate Total							
2 Estimate Total							
3 Estimate Total							
4 Estimate Total							
5 Estimate Total							
6 Estimate Total							
7 Estimate Total							

FOOD CHOICES

DAY ❶

Breakfast: _____

Lunch: _____

Dinner: _____

Snacks: _____

PHYSICAL ACTIVITY steps/miles/minutes: _____

description: _____

SPIRITUAL ACTIVITY

description: _____

FOOD CHOICES

DAY ❷

Breakfast: _____

Lunch: _____

Dinner: _____

Snacks: _____

PHYSICAL ACTIVITY   steps/miles/minutes:_____   **SPIRITUAL ACTIVITY**

description: _____   description: _____

_____   _____

FOOD CHOICES

DAY ❸

Breakfast: _____

Lunch: _____

Dinner: _____

Snacks: _____

PHYSICAL ACTIVITY   steps/miles/minutes:_____   **SPIRITUAL ACTIVITY**

description: _____   description: _____

_____   _____

FOOD CHOICES

DAY ❹

Breakfast: _____

Lunch: _____

Dinner: _____

Snacks: _____

PHYSICAL ACTIVITY   steps/miles/minutes:_____   **SPIRITUAL ACTIVITY**

description: _____   description: _____

_____   _____

FOOD CHOICES

DAY ❺

Breakfast: _____

Lunch: _____

Dinner: _____

Snacks: _____

PHYSICAL ACTIVITY   steps/miles/minutes:_____   **SPIRITUAL ACTIVITY**

description: _____   description: _____

_____   _____

FOOD CHOICES

DAY ❻

Breakfast: _____

Lunch: _____

Dinner: _____

Snacks: _____

PHYSICAL ACTIVITY   steps/miles/minutes:_____   **SPIRITUAL ACTIVITY**

description: _____   description: _____

_____   _____

FOOD CHOICES

DAY ❼

Breakfast: _____

Lunch: _____

Dinner: _____

Snacks: _____

PHYSICAL ACTIVITY   steps/miles/minutes:_____   **SPIRITUAL ACTIVITY**

description: _____   description: _____

_____   _____

LIVE IT TRACKER

Name: _____

Date: _____ Week #: _____

My activity goal for next week:
○ None   ○ <30 min/day   ○ 30-60 min/day

loss /gain _____ Calorie Range: _____

My week at a glance:
○ Great   ○ So-so   ○ Not so great

My food goal for next week: _____
_____

Activity level:
○ None   ○ <30 min/day   ○ 30-60 min/day

RECOMMENDED DAILY AMOUNT OF FOOD FROM EACH GROUP

GROUP	DAILY CALORIES							
....	1300-1400	1500-1600	1700-1800	1900-2000	2100-2200	2300-2400	2500-2600	2700-2800
Fruits	1.5 – 2 c.	1.5 – 2 c.	1.5 – 2 c.	2 – 2.5 c.	2 – 2.5 c.	2.5 – 3.5 c.	3.5 – 4.5 c.	3.5 – 4.5 c.
Vegetables	1.5 – 2 c.	2 – 2.5 c.	2.5 – 3 c.	2.5 – 3 c.	3 – 3.5 c.	3.5 – 4.5 c..	4.5 – 5 c.	4.5 – 5 c.
Grains	5 oz eq.	5-6 oz eq.	6-7 oz eq.	6-7 oz eq.	7-8 oz eq.	8-9 oz eq.	9-10 oz eq.	10-11 oz eq.
Dairy	2-3 c.	3 c.	3 c.	3 c.	3 c.	3 c.	3 c.	3 c.
Protein	4 oz eq.	5 oz eq.	5-5.5 oz eq.	5.5-6.5 oz eq.	6.5-7 oz eq.	7-7.5 oz eq.	7-7.5 oz eq.	7.5-8 oz eq.
Healthy Oils & Other Fats	4 tsp.	5 tsp.	5 tsp.	6 tsp.	6 tsp.	7 tsp.	8 tsp.	8 tsp.
Water & Super Beverages*	Women: 9 c. Men: 13 c.	Women: 9 c. Men: 13 c.	Women: 9 c. Men: 13 c.	Women: 9 c. Men: 13 c.	Women: 9 c. Men: 13 c.	Women: 9 c. Men: 13 c.	Women: 9 c. Men: 13 c.	Women: 9 c. Men: 13 c.

*May count up to 3 cups caffeinated tea or coffee toward goal

DAILY FOOD GROUP TRACKER

GROUP	FRUITS	VEGETABLES	GRAINS	PROTEIN	DAIRY	HEALTHY OILS & OTHER FATS	WATER & SUPER BEVERAGES
❶ Estimate Total							
❷ Estimate Total							
❸ Estimate Total							
❹ Estimate Total							
❺ Estimate Total							
❻ Estimate Total							
❼ Estimate Total							

FOOD CHOICES   DAY ❶

Breakfast: _____
Lunch: _____
Dinner: _____
Snacks: _____

PHYSICAL ACTIVITY   steps/miles/minutes: _____

description: _____
_____

SPIRITUAL ACTIVITY

description: _____
_____

FOOD CHOICES   DAY ❷

Breakfast: _____

Lunch: _____

Dinner: _____

Snacks: _____

PHYSICAL ACTIVITY   steps/miles/minutes:_____   **SPIRITUAL ACTIVITY**

description: _____   description: _____

FOOD CHOICES   DAY ❸

Breakfast: _____

Lunch: _____

Dinner: _____

Snacks: _____

PHYSICAL ACTIVITY   steps/miles/minutes:_____   **SPIRITUAL ACTIVITY**

description: _____   description: _____

FOOD CHOICES   DAY ❹

Breakfast: _____

Lunch: _____

Dinner: _____

Snacks: _____

PHYSICAL ACTIVITY   steps/miles/minutes:_____   **SPIRITUAL ACTIVITY**

description: _____   description: _____

FOOD CHOICES   DAY ❺

Breakfast: _____

Lunch: _____

Dinner: _____

Snacks: _____

PHYSICAL ACTIVITY   steps/miles/minutes:_____   **SPIRITUAL ACTIVITY**

description: _____   description: _____

FOOD CHOICES   DAY ❻

Breakfast: _____

Lunch: _____

Dinner: _____

Snacks: _____

PHYSICAL ACTIVITY   steps/miles/minutes:_____   **SPIRITUAL ACTIVITY**

description: _____   description: _____

FOOD CHOICES   DAY ❼

Breakfast: _____

Lunch: _____

Dinner: _____

Snacks: _____

PHYSICAL ACTIVITY   steps/miles/minutes:_____   **SPIRITUAL ACTIVITY**

description: _____   description: _____

LIVE IT TRACKER

Name: _____

Date: _____ Week #: _____

My activity goal for next week:
○ None   ○ <30 min/day   ○ 30-60 min/day

loss / gain _____ Calorie Range: _____

My week at a glance:
○ Great   ○ So-so   ○ Not so great

My food goal for next week: _____
_____

Activity level:
○ None   ○ <30 min/day   ○ 30-60 min/day

RECOMMENDED DAILY AMOUNT OF FOOD FROM EACH GROUP

GROUP	DAILY CALORIES							
	1300-1400	1500-1600	1700-1800	1900-2000	2100-2200	2300-2400	2500-2600	2700-2800
Fruits	1.5 – 2 c.	1.5 – 2 c.	1.5 – 2 c.	2 – 2.5 c.	2 – 2.5 c.	2.5 – 3.5 c.	3.5 – 4.5 c.	3.5 – 4.5 c.
Vegetables	1.5 – 2 c.	2 – 2.5 c.	2.5 – 3 c.	2.5 – 3 c.	3 – 3.5 c.	3.5 – 4.5 c..	4.5 – 5 c.	4.5 – 5 c.
Grains	5 oz eq.	5-6 oz eq.	6-7 oz eq.	6-7 oz eq.	7-8 oz eq.	8-9 oz eq.	9-10 oz eq.	10-11 oz eq.
Dairy	2-3 c.	3 c.	3 c.	3 c.	3 c.	3 c.	3 c.	3 c.
Protein	4 oz eq.	5 oz eq.	5-5.5 oz eq.	5.5-6.5 oz eq.	6.5-7 oz eq.	7-7.5 oz eq.	7-7.5 oz eq.	7.5-8 oz eq.
Healthy Oils & Other Fats	4 tsp.	5 tsp.	5 tsp.	6 tsp.	6 tsp.	7 tsp.	8 tsp.	8 tsp.
Water & Super Beverages*	Women: 9 c. Men: 13 c.	Women: 9 c. Men: 13 c.	Women: 9 c. Men: 13 c.	Women: 9 c. Men: 13 c.	Women: 9 c. Men: 13 c.	Women: 9 c. Men: 13 c.	Women: 9 c. Men: 13 c.	Women: 9 c. Men: 13 c.

*May count up to 3 cups caffeinated tea or coffee toward goal

DAILY FOOD GROUP TRACKER

GROUP	FRUITS	VEGETABLES	GRAINS	PROTEIN	DAIRY	HEALTHY OILS & OTHER FATS	WATER & SUPER BEVERAGES
① Estimate Total							
② Estimate Total							
③ Estimate Total							
④ Estimate Total							
⑤ Estimate Total							
⑥ Estimate Total							
⑦ Estimate Total							

FOOD CHOICES   DAY ❶

Breakfast: _____
Lunch: _____
Dinner: _____
Snacks: _____

PHYSICAL ACTIVITY steps/miles/minutes: _____

description: _____
_____

SPIRITUAL ACTIVITY

description: _____
_____

FOOD CHOICES **DAY ②**

Breakfast: _____

Lunch: _____

Dinner: _____

Snacks: _____

PHYSICAL ACTIVITY   steps/miles/minutes: _____   SPIRITUAL ACTIVITY

description: _____   description: _____

FOOD CHOICES **DAY ③**

Breakfast: _____

Lunch: _____

Dinner: _____

Snacks: _____

PHYSICAL ACTIVITY   steps/miles/minutes: _____   SPIRITUAL ACTIVITY

description: _____   description: _____

FOOD CHOICES **DAY ④**

Breakfast: _____

Lunch: _____

Dinner: _____

Snacks: _____

PHYSICAL ACTIVITY   steps/miles/minutes: _____   SPIRITUAL ACTIVITY

description: _____   description: _____

FOOD CHOICES **DAY ⑤**

Breakfast: _____

Lunch: _____

Dinner: _____

Snacks: _____

PHYSICAL ACTIVITY   steps/miles/minutes: _____   SPIRITUAL ACTIVITY

description: _____   description: _____

FOOD CHOICES **DAY ⑥**

Breakfast: _____

Lunch: _____

Dinner: _____

Snacks: _____

PHYSICAL ACTIVITY   steps/miles/minutes: _____   SPIRITUAL ACTIVITY

description: _____   description: _____

FOOD CHOICES **DAY ⑦**

Breakfast: _____

Lunch: _____

Dinner: _____

Snacks: _____

PHYSICAL ACTIVITY   steps/miles/minutes: _____   SPIRITUAL ACTIVITY

description: _____   description: _____

Name: _____

Date: _____ Week #: _____

My activity goal for next week:
○ None   ○ <30 min/day   ○ 30-60 min/day

loss/gain _____   Calorie Range: _____

My week at a glance:
○ Great   ○ So-so   ○ Not so great

Activity level:
○ None   ○ <30 min/day   ○ 30-60 min/day

My food goal for next week: _____
_____

RECOMMENDED DAILY AMOUNT OF FOOD FROM EACH GROUP

GROUP	DAILY CALORIES							
....	1300-1400	1500-1600	1700-1800	1900-2000	2100-2200	2300-2400	2500-2600	2700-2800
Fruits	1.5 – 2 c.	1.5 – 2 c.	1.5 – 2 c.	2 – 2.5 c.	2 – 2.5 c.	2.5 – 3.5 c.	3.5 – 4.5 c.	3.5 – 4.5 c.
Vegetables	1.5 – 2 c.	2 – 2.5 c.	2.5 – 3 c.	2.5 – 3 c.	3 – 3.5 c.	3.5 – 4.5 c..	4.5 – 5 c.	4.5 – 5 c.
Grains	5 oz eq.	5-6 oz eq.	6-7 oz eq.	6-7 oz eq.	7-8 oz eq.	8-9 oz eq.	9-10 oz eq.	10-11 oz eq.
Dairy	2-3 c.	3 c.	3 c.	3 c.	3 c.	3 c.	3 c.	3 c.
Protein	4 oz eq.	5 oz eq.	5-5.5 oz eq.	5.5-6.5 oz eq.	6.5-7 oz eq.	7-7.5 oz eq.	7-7.5 oz eq.	7.5-8 oz eq.
Healthy Oils & Other Fats	4 tsp.	5 tsp.	5 tsp.	6 tsp.	6 tsp.	7 tsp.	8 tsp.	8 tsp.
Water & Super Beverages*	Women: 9 c. Men: 13 c.	Women: 9 c. Men: 13 c.	Women: 9 c. Men: 13 c.	Women: 9 c. Men: 13 c.	Women: 9 c. Men: 13 c.	Women: 9 c. Men: 13 c.	Women: 9 c. Men: 13 c.	Women: 9 c. Men: 13 c.

*May count up to 3 cups caffeinated tea or coffee toward goal

DAILY FOOD GROUP TRACKER

GROUP	FRUITS	VEGETABLES	GRAINS	PROTEIN	DAIRY	HEALTHY OILS & OTHER FATS	WATER & SUPER BEVERAGES
1 Estimate Total							
2 Estimate Total							
3 Estimate Total							
4 Estimate Total							
5 Estimate Total							
6 Estimate Total							
7 Estimate Total							

FOOD CHOICES   DAY 1

Breakfast: _____
Lunch: _____
Dinner: _____
Snacks: _____

PHYSICAL ACTIVITY   steps/miles/minutes: _____

description: _____
_____

SPIRITUAL ACTIVITY

description: _____
_____

FOOD CHOICES

DAY ❷

Breakfast: _____

Lunch: _____

Dinner: _____

Snacks: _____

PHYSICAL ACTIVITY steps/miles/minutes: _____

description: _____

SPIRITUAL ACTIVITY

description: _____

FOOD CHOICES

DAY ❸

Breakfast: _____

Lunch: _____

Dinner: _____

Snacks: _____

PHYSICAL ACTIVITY steps/miles/minutes: _____

description: _____

SPIRITUAL ACTIVITY

description: _____

FOOD CHOICES

DAY ❹

Breakfast: _____

Lunch: _____

Dinner: _____

Snacks: _____

PHYSICAL ACTIVITY steps/miles/minutes: _____

description: _____

SPIRITUAL ACTIVITY

description: _____

FOOD CHOICES

DAY ❺

Breakfast: _____

Lunch: _____

Dinner: _____

Snacks: _____

PHYSICAL ACTIVITY steps/miles/minutes: _____

description: _____

SPIRITUAL ACTIVITY

description: _____

FOOD CHOICES

DAY ❻

Breakfast: _____

Lunch: _____

Dinner: _____

Snacks: _____

PHYSICAL ACTIVITY steps/miles/minutes: _____

description: _____

SPIRITUAL ACTIVITY

description: _____

FOOD CHOICES

DAY ❼

Breakfast: _____

Lunch: _____

Dinner: _____

Snacks: _____

PHYSICAL ACTIVITY steps/miles/minutes: _____

description: _____

SPIRITUAL ACTIVITY

description: _____

LIVE IT TRACKER

Name: _____

Date: _____ Week #: _____

My activity goal for next week:
○ None ○ <30 min/day ○ 30-60 min/day

loss / gain _____ Calorie Range: _____

My week at a glance:
○ Great ○ So-so ○ Not so great

My food goal for next week: _____

Activity level:
○ None ○ <30 min/day ○ 30-60 min/day

RECOMMENDED DAILY AMOUNT OF FOOD FROM EACH GROUP

GROUP	DAILY CALORIES							
....	1300-1400	1500-1600	1700-1800	1900-2000	2100-2200	2300-2400	2500-2600	2700-2800
Fruits	1.5 – 2 c.	1.5 – 2 c.	1.5 – 2 c.	2 – 2.5 c.	2 – 2.5 c.	2.5 – 3.5 c.	3.5 – 4.5 c.	3.5 – 4.5 c.
Vegetables	1.5 – 2 c.	2 – 2.5 c.	2.5 – 3 c.	2.5 – 3 c.	3 – 3.5 c.	3.5 – 4.5 c..	4.5 – 5 c.	4.5 – 5 c.
Grains	5 oz eq.	5-6 oz eq.	6-7 oz eq.	6-7 oz eq.	7-8 oz eq.	8-9 oz eq.	9-10 oz eq.	10-11 oz eq.
Dairy	2-3 c.	3 c.	3 c.	3 c.	3 c.	3 c.	3 c.	3 c.
Protein	4 oz eq.	5 oz eq.	5-5.5 oz eq.	5.5-6.5 oz eq.	6.5-7 oz eq.	7-7.5 oz eq.	7-7.5 oz eq.	7.5-8 oz eq.
Healthy Oils & Other Fats	4 tsp.	5 tsp.	5 tsp.	6 tsp.	6 tsp.	7 tsp.	8 tsp.	8 tsp.
Water & Super Beverages*	Women: 9 c. Men: 13 c.	Women: 9 c. Men: 13 c.	Women: 9 c. Men: 13 c.	Women: 9 c. Men: 13 c.	Women: 9 c. Men: 13 c.	Women: 9 c. Men: 13 c.	Women: 9 c. Men: 13 c.	Women: 9 c. Men: 13 c.

*May count up to 3 cups caffeinated tea or coffee toward goal

DAILY FOOD GROUP TRACKER

GROUP	FRUITS	VEGETABLES	GRAINS	PROTEIN	DAIRY	HEALTHY OILS & OTHER FATS	WATER & SUPER BEVERAGES
❶ Estimate Total							
❷ Estimate Total							
❸ Estimate Total							
❹ Estimate Total							
❺ Estimate Total							
❻ Estimate Total							
❼ Estimate Total							

FOOD CHOICES   DAY ❶

Breakfast: _____

Lunch: _____

Dinner: _____

Snacks: _____

PHYSICAL ACTIVITY   steps/miles/minutes: _____

description: _____

SPIRITUAL ACTIVITY

description: _____

FOOD CHOICES — DAY ❷

Breakfast: _____
Lunch: _____
Dinner: _____
Snacks: _____

PHYSICAL ACTIVITY   steps/miles/minutes: _____

description: _____

SPIRITUAL ACTIVITY

description: _____

FOOD CHOICES — DAY ❸

Breakfast: _____
Lunch: _____
Dinner: _____
Snacks: _____

PHYSICAL ACTIVITY   steps/miles/minutes: _____

description: _____

SPIRITUAL ACTIVITY

description: _____

FOOD CHOICES — DAY ❹

Breakfast: _____
Lunch: _____
Dinner: _____
Snacks: _____

PHYSICAL ACTIVITY   steps/miles/minutes: _____

description: _____

SPIRITUAL ACTIVITY

description: _____

FOOD CHOICES — DAY ❺

Breakfast: _____
Lunch: _____
Dinner: _____
Snacks: _____

PHYSICAL ACTIVITY   steps/miles/minutes: _____

description: _____

SPIRITUAL ACTIVITY

description: _____

FOOD CHOICES — DAY ❻

Breakfast: _____
Lunch: _____
Dinner: _____
Snacks: _____

PHYSICAL ACTIVITY   steps/miles/minutes: _____

description: _____

SPIRITUAL ACTIVITY

description: _____

FOOD CHOICES — DAY ❼

Breakfast: _____
Lunch: _____
Dinner: _____
Snacks: _____

PHYSICAL ACTIVITY   steps/miles/minutes: _____

description: _____

SPIRITUAL ACTIVITY

description: _____

LIVE IT TRACKER

Name: _____

Date: _____ Week #: _____

My activity goal for next week:
○ None   ○ <30 min/day   ○ 30-60 min/day

loss/gain _____ Calorie Range: _____

My week at a glance:
○ Great   ○ So-so   ○ Not so great

My food goal for next week: _____

Activity level:
○ None   ○ <30 min/day   ○ 30-60 min/day

RECOMMENDED DAILY AMOUNT OF FOOD FROM EACH GROUP

GROUP	DAILY CALORIES							
	1300-1400	1500-1600	1700-1800	1900-2000	2100-2200	2300-2400	2500-2600	2700-2800
Fruits	1.5 – 2 c.	1.5 – 2 c.	1.5 – 2 c.	2 – 2.5 c.	2 – 2.5 c.	2.5 – 3.5 c.	3.5 – 4.5 c.	3.5 – 4.5 c.
Vegetables	1.5 – 2 c.	2 – 2.5 c.	2.5 – 3 c.	2.5 – 3 c.	3 – 3.5 c.	3.5 – 4.5 c..	4.5 – 5 c.	4.5 – 5 c.
Grains	5 oz eq.	5-6 oz eq.	6-7 oz eq.	6-7 oz eq.	7-8 oz eq.	8-9 oz eq.	9-10 oz eq.	10-11 oz eq.
Dairy	2-3 c.	3 c.	3 c.	3 c.	3 c.	3 c.	3 c.	3 c.
Protein	4 oz eq.	5 oz eq.	5-5.5 oz eq.	5.5-6.5 oz eq.	6.5-7 oz eq.	7-7.5 oz eq.	7-7.5 oz eq.	7.5-8 oz eq.
Healthy Oils & Other Fats	4 tsp.	5 tsp.	5 tsp.	6 tsp.	6 tsp.	7 tsp.	8 tsp.	8 tsp.
Water & Super Beverages*	Women: 9 c. Men: 13 c.	Women: 9 c. Men: 13 c.	Women: 9 c. Men: 13 c.	Women: 9 c. Men: 13 c.	Women: 9 c. Men: 13 c.	Women: 9 c. Men: 13 c.	Women: 9 c. Men: 13 c.	Women: 9 c. Men: 13 c.

*May count up to 3 cups caffeinated tea or coffee toward goal

DAILY FOOD GROUP TRACKER

GROUP	FRUITS	VEGETABLES	GRAINS	PROTEIN	DAIRY	HEALTHY OILS & OTHER FATS	WATER & SUPER BEVERAGES
① Estimate Total							
② Estimate Total							
③ Estimate Total							
④ Estimate Total							
⑤ Estimate Total							
⑥ Estimate Total							
⑦ Estimate Total							

FOOD CHOICES

DAY ❶

Breakfast: _____
Lunch: _____
Dinner: _____
Snacks: _____

PHYSICAL ACTIVITY   steps/miles/minutes: _____

description: _____

SPIRITUAL ACTIVITY

description: _____

FOOD CHOICES
DAY ❷

Breakfast: _____
Lunch: _____
Dinner: _____
Snacks: _____

PHYSICAL ACTIVITY steps/miles/minutes:_____

description: _____

SPIRITUAL ACTIVITY

description: _____

FOOD CHOICES
DAY ❸

Breakfast: _____
Lunch: _____
Dinner: _____
Snacks: _____

PHYSICAL ACTIVITY steps/miles/minutes:_____

description: _____

SPIRITUAL ACTIVITY

description: _____

FOOD CHOICES
DAY ❹

Breakfast: _____
Lunch: _____
Dinner: _____
Snacks: _____

PHYSICAL ACTIVITY steps/miles/minutes:_____

description: _____

SPIRITUAL ACTIVITY

description: _____

FOOD CHOICES
DAY ❺

Breakfast: _____
Lunch: _____
Dinner: _____
Snacks: _____

PHYSICAL ACTIVITY steps/miles/minutes:_____

description: _____

SPIRITUAL ACTIVITY

description: _____

FOOD CHOICES
DAY ❻

Breakfast: _____
Lunch: _____
Dinner: _____
Snacks: _____

PHYSICAL ACTIVITY steps/miles/minutes:_____

description: _____

SPIRITUAL ACTIVITY

description: _____

FOOD CHOICES
DAY ❼

Breakfast: _____
Lunch: _____
Dinner: _____
Snacks: _____

PHYSICAL ACTIVITY steps/miles/minutes:_____

description: _____

SPIRITUAL ACTIVITY

description: _____